Keto
Cookbook

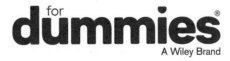

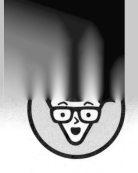

Keto Cookbook

by Rami Abrams and Vicky Abrams

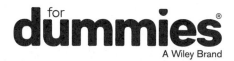

A Wiley Brand

Keto Cookbook For Dummies®

Published by: **John Wiley & Sons, Inc.,** 111 River Street, Hoboken, NJ 07030-5774, www.wiley.com

Copyright © 2023 by John Wiley & Sons, Inc., Hoboken, New Jersey

Published simultaneously in Canada

No part of this publication may be reproduced, stored in a retrieval system or transmitted in any form or by any means, electronic, mechanical, photocopying, recording, scanning or otherwise, except as permitted under Sections 107 or 108 of the 1976 United States Copyright Act, without the prior written permission of the Publisher. Requests to the Publisher for permission should be addressed to the Permissions Department, John Wiley & Sons, Inc., 111 River Street, Hoboken, NJ 07030, (201) 748-6011, fax (201) 748-6008, or online at http://www.wiley.com/go/permissions.

Trademarks: Wiley, For Dummies, the Dummies Man logo, Dummies.com, Making Everything Easier, and related trade dress are trademarks or registered trademarks of John Wiley & Sons, Inc. and may not be used without written permission. All other trademarks are the property of their respective owners. John Wiley & Sons, Inc. is not associated with any product or vendor mentioned in this book.

LIMIT OF LIABILITY/DISCLAIMER OF WARRANTY: WHILE THE PUBLISHER AND AUTHORS HAVE USED THEIR BEST EFFORTS IN PREPARING THIS WORK, THEY MAKE NO REPRESENTATIONS OR WARRANTIES WITH RESPECT TO THE ACCURACY OR COMPLETENESS OF THE CONTENTS OF THIS WORK AND SPECIFICALLY DISCLAIM ALL WARRANTIES, INCLUDING WITHOUT LIMITATION ANY IMPLIED WARRANTIES OF MERCHANTABILITY OR FITNESS FOR A PARTICULAR PURPOSE. NO WARRANTY MAY BE CREATED OR EXTENDED BY SALES REPRESENTATIVES, WRITTEN SALES MATERIALS OR PROMOTIONAL STATEMENTS FOR THIS WORK. THE FACT THAT AN ORGANIZATION, WEBSITE, OR PRODUCT IS REFERRED TO IN THIS WORK AS A CITATION AND/OR POTENTIAL SOURCE OF FURTHER INFORMATION DOES NOT MEAN THAT THE PUBLISHER AND AUTHORS ENDORSE THE INFORMATION OR SERVICES THE ORGANIZATION, WEBSITE, OR PRODUCT MAY PROVIDE OR RECOMMENDATIONS IT MAY MAKE. THIS WORK IS SOLD WITH THE UNDERSTANDING THAT THE PUBLISHER IS NOT ENGAGED IN RENDERING PROFESSIONAL SERVICES. THE ADVICE AND STRATEGIES CONTAINED HEREIN MAY NOT BE SUITABLE FOR YOUR SITUATION. YOU SHOULD CONSULT WITH A SPECIALIST WHERE APPROPRIATE. FURTHER, READERS SHOULD BE AWARE THAT WEBSITES LISTED IN THIS WORK MAY HAVE CHANGED OR DISAPPEARED BETWEEN WHEN THIS WORK WAS WRITTEN AND WHEN IT IS READ. NEITHER THE PUBLISHER NOR AUTHORS SHALL BE LIABLE FOR ANY LOSS OF PROFIT OR ANY OTHER COMMERCIAL DAMAGES, INCLUDING BUT NOT LIMITED TO SPECIAL, INCIDENTAL, CONSEQUENTIAL, OR OTHER DAMAGES.

For general information on our other products and services, please contact our Customer Care Department within the U.S. at 877-762-2974, outside the U.S. at 317-572-3993, or fax 317-572-4002. For technical support, please visit https://hub.wiley.com/community/support/dummies.

Wiley publishes in a variety of print and electronic formats and by print-on-demand. Some material included with standard print versions of this book may not be included in e-books or in print-on-demand. If this book refers to media such as a CD or DVD that is not included in the version you purchased, you may download this material at http://booksupport.wiley.com. For more information about Wiley products, visit www.wiley.com.

Library of Congress Control Number: 2023930251

ISBN 978-1-394-16877-4 (pbk); ISBN 978-1-394-16878-1 (ebk); ISBN 978-1-394-16879-8 (ebk)

SKY10041785_012623

Contents at a Glance

Recipes at a Glance

Salads

Lunches

Fish Dinners

Meat Dinners

Vegetarian Breakfasts

Vegetarian Appetizers

Vegetarian Lunches

Vegetarian Dinners

Air Fryer Recipes

Instant Pot and Slow Cooker Meals

Meal Prep for the Week

Drinks

Snacks

Desserts

Table of Contents

Introduction

Are you looking to lose a significant amount of weight in a relatively short period? Tired of extreme diets that restrict calories to near-starvation levels, only to put back on those pounds you worked so hard to lose when you get back to eating normally? Is your doctor telling you to improve your cholesterol levels or watch your blood sugar? It may be surprising to discover that you can achieve your weight-loss goals and become healthier by changing what and how you eat. The standard American diet (which we think is very appropriately abbreviated as SAD) is based on consuming high levels of carbohydrates daily and avoiding most fats. Unfortunately for many Americans and much of the world, we've been led to believe that eating tons of carbs is excellent for your health while fat makes you fat. As a result, we've reached the highest-ever levels in history (by percentage of the population) of obesity, prediabetes, type 2 diabetes, and heart disease.

We're going to show you a better approach to eating that focuses on low amounts of carbohydrates and high levels of fat. This approach is known as the ketogenic diet (or keto for short).

About This Book

We've written this book so you can find information quickly and easily. Each chapter focuses on a specific aspect of the ketogenic diet and outlines how to make the transition, accentuating benefits while minimizing downsides and structuring your diet and lifestyle to create your best "you." There are specific details and practical tips, but you don't have to read the book from front to back. Feel free to skip around, browse the sections that you find interesting, and follow where your questions take you.

Reading this entire book isn't necessary to experience a successful keto journey. We've designed it as a resource you can refer to continually. Make notes in the margins, jot down additional resources or recipe adjustments, and highlight the most applicable information to your unique situation. In short, make this book a reflection of your ketogenic exploration and customize it to fit you!

Throughout the book, you'll notice sidebars or text in gray boxes. If you're short on time, you can skip that text — they're interesting but not essential to understanding the topic.

In the recipes, the oven and internal meat thermometer temperatures are in Fahrenheit, but the Appendix can help you convert the temperatures to Celsius, if needed.

Finally, within this book, you may note that some web addresses break across two lines of text. If you're reading this book in print and want to visit one of these web pages, key in the web address exactly as it's noted in the text, pretending that the line break doesn't exist. If you're reading this as an e-book, you've got it easy — click the web address to be taken directly to the web page.

Foolish Assumptions

As we wrote this book, we made the following assumptions about you:

» You want to change your diet, lose weight, improve your fitness, or manage some medical condition.

» You have control over your and your family's food choices and want to encourage your family to enjoy a healthy, low-carb lifestyle.

» You want to minimize processed and unhealthy junk foods and maximize wholesome food choices to feel younger, healthier, and happier.

» You're interested in finding out how food choices affect you physically and mentally, but you don't want to get bogged down in all the scientific jargon. You want a summary of what you need to know in plain English.

» You're open to making lifestyle changes — avoiding certain foods, making sleep a priority, adopting a fitness program — to enhance your quality of life.

Icons Used in This Book

Throughout this book, we use *icons* (little pictures in the margin) to draw your attention to certain kinds of information. Here are the icons we use, and what they mean:

TIP

Whenever you see the Tip icon, you can be sure to find a nugget of information that will make your life on keto easier in some way — big or small.

REMEMBER

This book is a reference, which means you don't have to commit it to memory and there won't be a test on Friday. However, sometimes we do tell you something that's so important that you'll want to file it away for future use, and when we do, we mark that information with the Remember icon.

WARNING

When you see the Warning icon, beware! We're letting you know about a pitfall or danger that you'll want to avoid.

Finally, we use a little tomato icon (🍅) to highlight vegetarian recipes in the Recipes in This Chapter lists, as well as in the Recipes at a Glance at the front of this book.

Beyond the Book

In addition to the book you have in your hand, you can access some helpful extra content online. Check out the free Cheat Sheet, which includes the following:

>> Getting Started with Keto Checklist

>> Keto and Low-Carb Food List

>> Counting Net Carbs

>> Using Keto Baking and Cooking Alternatives

>> Fast Keto Snacks List

>> Keto-Friendly Alcohol List

You can access it by going to www.dummies.com and entering "Keto Cookbook For Dummies" in the Search box.

Where to Go from Here

You can read this book from beginning to end, or you can use the table of contents and index to locate the topics you're most interested in right now. If you're not sure where to start, you can't go wrong with Chapter 1. If you'd rather start cooking, head to Part 2 or use the Recipes at a Glance at the start of the book to find the kind of recipe you're looking for, from breakfasts to desserts. If you're curious about fasting, Chapter 7 is for you. And if you'd just like a quick reminder of ten great benefits of being in ketosis, head to Chapter 26. Wherever you start, we hope the keto diet is as rewarding for you as it is for us!

1

Succeeding with the Keto Lifestyle

IN THIS PART . . .

Discover what the keto diet is all about.

Consider the benefits of the keto diet.

Make your kitchen keto-friendly.

Understand which foods are keto.

Identify macronutrients and how they affect you.

Go out to eat while staying keto.

Try out intermittent fasting for a metabolism boost.

Get over any obstacles.

Chapter **1**

Embracing Keto for Your Well-Being

The keto diet has exploded in popularity in the last 10 years, but other than it being a great way to lose weight, what do you really know about this popular diet? Is it really a healthy way to lose weight? Is there more to it than eating bacon and eggs? We are here to help you figure out whether the keto diet is right for you and to teach you the basic steps of safely and effectively following a keto lifestyle. In this chapter, we introduce the core concepts of the keto diet.

Exploring the Keto Diet

The ketogenic diet (also known as the keto diet) is a tried-and-true method to improve your health by working with your body through your dietary practices. The keto lifestyle can help you

>> Have more energy

>> Quickly lose weight

>> Improve your heart health

>> Improve your ability to focus

Though it has become more popular recently, the keto diet has been used for almost a hundred years to prevent disease and help the body heal. That's an amazing track record for any diet! The benefits of the keto diet are just that good.

So, what exactly is the keto diet? The keto diet involves eating foods that are

>> High in fat

>> Moderate in protein

>> Very low in carbohydrates

Easily digested carbohydrates fuel weight gain and cause unhealthy spikes in blood sugar. Throughout a lifetime, this can really take a toll on your health.

The keto diet puts your body into a metabolic state called *ketosis,* when your body uses fats, rather than carbs, for fuel. You'll learn everything to know about ketosis in Chapter 2!

There are many misconceptions about nutrition in general, and the keto diet especially. The keto lifestyle is much more than "bacon, eggs, and cheese" — although you can eat bacon and cheese as much as you'd like! It won't clog your arteries or make you fat, nor will it increase your cholesterol levels if you follow a whole-food-based keto lifestyle.

For example, one of the most common misconceptions is that fat is bad for you. Fat is actually very good for you, keeps you feeling fuller longer, helps you lose weight, and improves your health over the long term.

Additionally, you don't need to eat many carbs as part of a healthy lifestyle. For many reasons, your body stores fat — and not carbs — for energy. Fat provides 9 calories (energy) per gram, while carbs only provide 4 calories per gram! Fat is a slow, continuous energy source compared to carbs, which are glucose at the most basic level. Carbs spike blood glucose and require your body to produce insulin to then reduce blood glucose to safe levels.

Eating a whole range of low-carb foods is the key to a healthy lifestyle. The best part is that keto is a flexible diet with multiple variations to fit your lifestyle and goals! It isn't a one-size-fits-all plan.

There are several different variations of the keto diet. Take a look at each one to see which version fits your personal goals and the way you prefer to eat.

Standard ketogenic diet

The standard ketogenic diet is the most basic, straightforward version of the keto diet. It is the most researched and has been around the longest of the various types of keto diets. It clearly breaks down the sources of your daily calorie intake so you can easily start your keto diet. Here is what to eat on the standard keto diet:

>> **Fat:** 70 percent of your daily calories

>> **Protein:** 25 percent of your daily calories

>> **Carbohydrates:** 5 percent of your daily calories

On this diet, you generally eat about 25 to 30 grams of carbohydrates per day; however, this number is flexible. This amount of carbs is about one-fifth to one-tenth of what many Americans eat per day, so you can start to see why making such a radical change from a carb-based diet to a fat-based one has a massive, positive impact on your health and energy levels.

REMEMBER

The standard ketogenic diet's ratio is 70:25:5 in terms of calories from fat, protein, and carbs as shown in Figure 1-1. You should aim for up to 30 grams of carbs per day.

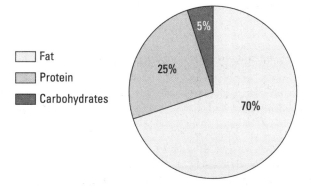

FIGURE 1-1:
Standard keto diet percentages.

Targeted ketogenic diet

The targeted keto diet is often used by athletes because it's more flexible when it comes to carb intake. This diet allows more carbs when you know you will be especially active. The extra carbs are burned immediately during your intense workouts, allowing you to stay in ketosis but still get a bit of extra energy.

Keep in mind that this is not a free pass to eat as many carbs as you want. About 25 to 30 grams of easily digestible carbs are okay about 30 to 45 minutes before a hard workout like high-intensity interval training (HIIT), 30 minute or longer jogs, hour or longer of weight lifting. After that exercise is over, you go right back to the regular keto diet. Remember to count the total number of calories (including your pre-workout carbs) when coming up with your daily energy intake.

REMEMBER

It is important to eat only enough carbs to fuel your workout so your body returns to burning fats after you exercise. It's a good idea to get your body adjusted to the standard keto diet for a few months before switching to a targeted keto diet.

Cyclical ketogenic diet

The cyclical keto diet is another flexible version of keto that caters to athletes. It allows athletes to up their carb intake for a short time to "fuel" themselves for a performance. Once the big event is over, you return to the standard keto diet. Although this may kick you out of ketosis, the intense activity ensures that all those extra carbs are burned.

The cyclical keto diet is also good for people who need cheat days. You can go 5 days on the keto diet and then cheat a little on the weekends. However, it is important to remember that on those cheat days, you still shouldn't binge on carbs. It can be tough on the body to go from no carbs to high carbs. Instead, opt for a low-carb diet on cheat days, ranging from 150 to 200 grams of carbs rather than the lower quantities typically allowed on the keto diet. You won't be in ketosis on the cheat days, but it can sometimes help people who really miss the carbs.

TIP

Consider the cyclical keto diet if any of the following applies to you:

>> **You are an elite bodybuilder or short-distance sprinter who has been training for years.** And you've noticed drops in your performance and realize that you need more carbs to fuel your intense level of activity.

>> **You are otherwise healthy and don't have any metabolic reasons to believe that "carb loading" will affect your health.** If you notice an improvement in blood pressure or blood sugar levels, cyclical keto is *not* for you because you may lose all your gains when you cycle out of ketosis.

>> **You work out intensely and on a specific schedule.** Your high-carb days should coincide with the days that you're at the gym. Also, you need to be able to cycle in and out of ketosis by completely depleting the excess carbs you consume on your workout days and then switch back into a keto diet on non-carb-loading days.

Generally, cyclical keto helps with gains for anaerobic exercises including 100-meter sprints, low-rep maximums (four to six) for weightlifters, or CrossFit circuits.

High-protein ketogenic diet

The high-protein keto diet is just as it sounds — higher in protein! Here is a quick look at the breakdown of a high-protein keto diet:

>> **Fat:** 60 percent of your daily calories

>> **Protein:** 35 percent of your daily calories

>> **Carbohydrate:** 5 percent of your daily calories

This version of the keto diet is great for anyone who is concerned about losing muscle mass or not gaining enough while working out consistently. Adding protein is a great way to help gain muscle and remain in ketosis. Keto is considered a *muscle neutral* diet, meaning you don't really gain or lose muscle because your body is efficiently utilizing the fat you eat and stored fat even while at a caloric deficit. This is another benefit of keto because on high-carb diets, when in a caloric deficit, your body more readily taps into muscle protein for the remainder energy, so you lose muscle in addition to fat.

Keep in mind, it's difficult, but possible, to get kicked out of ketosis if you go higher than the recommended 35 percent of calories from protein (see Figure 1-2). Remember to eat a range of proteins that are nutritious and filling.

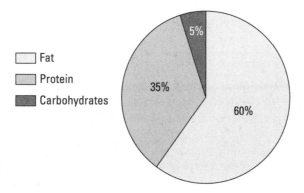

FIGURE 1-2:
High-protein keto diet percentages.

Setting Realistic Expectations on Keto

Before you dive into the keto diet, you should be sure that it is the right fit for you. Having realistic expectations is key to your success. While the keto diet can be adapted to fit the needs of almost everyone, you should fully understand the benefits and the few side effects of the diet (which we go over in Chapter 2). Keep reading to really assess whether keto is right for you.

Use SMART goals to set yourself up for success

It's a good idea to set goals on any diet. We specifically like to use SMART goals. SMART is an acronym for

» **S**pecific

» **M**easurable

» **A**chievable

» **R**elevant

» **T**ime-based

Goals should be specific. For example, a nonspecific goal would be to "lose weight" or "get in better shape." You could lose two pounds and technically fulfill both of those goals, but you wouldn't really hit your goal. An example of a specific goal is this: "I want to lose 10 pounds of fat by June 1st."

Instead of "losing some weight," it's better to strive for a measurable goal like losing 10 pounds. You can also strive for completing a sporting event, such as a marathon, or a defined achievement, like benching or squatting a certain weight.

Another reason we often fail to achieve our goals is because the goals we set are not attainable, at least for that moment in our lives. Every person's body is unique; trying to achieve the body of a supermodel or bodybuilder isn't possible for most people, and that's totally fine! Use your goals to set yourself up for success. If last week you jogged for 10 minutes a day, next week try to jog for 12 or 15 minutes. If last week you worked out 3 days of the week, this week try to work out for 4 days. Small, attainable goals and improvements keep you motivated.

Your goals should be relevant to what's important for you. If you're trying to build muscle, and you set yourself a goal to run a marathon by a specific date, that most likely will not get you to the image of success you've painted in your mind, even if you accomplish your goal. It's crucial to create goals that are relevant to achieving the success you really want.

Finally, make your goals time-based. Try to give yourself enough time to make them happen, but put some pressure on yourself. You may have specific goals that are well-defined and measurable; they're attainable and very relevant to your definition of success. If you say that you'll accomplish all of that "someday," however, you'll never hit the mark. You need to be pushed to meet your goals by a deadline, giving you a sense of urgency that you must keep pressing every day or you won't make it there.

The elements of SMART work together to create goals that are well-planned, clear, and trackable. This strategy completely applies to the keto diet.

Define your weight-loss goals or maintenance targets

So, what are your goals when it comes to the keto diet? Do you want to lose weight quickly and keep it off? Are you looking to decrease your risk of diabetes? Are you trying to improve your daily energy levels? The keto diet can help with each of those goals, but you need to define your personal goals before you jump into the keto lifestyle.

Having achievable targets helps you stick to your keto diet. When you have something you are working toward, you are more likely to continue with your keto diet commitment and achieve success. If you want to get healthy and stay that way, you can with keto!

REMEMBER

The keto diet may be for you if you are ready to commit to changing your diet and health in a positive way. Commitment and drive are essential to your success!

Measure your success

Success means something different for everyone; however, there are some telltale signs of success when you're on the keto diet that you'll recognize as you embark on your journey.

The first and largely most popular metric is weight loss.

In the first week, you'll likely lose 7 to 10 pounds. It's very important to understand that this isn't all fat. In fact, it's mostly water weight. It looks great and feels great on the scale and is a huge motivational boost to continue with the diet.

The reason you lose so much water weight initially is due to your body burning through *glycogen* (glucose stored in your muscles) and dumping all the water your muscles hold. After the first week, the weight loss will slow down but will be primarily fat loss, so keep on going!

As you lose weight, sometimes you may not see it in the mirror or even on the scale! There are a variety of reasons why this could happen, including the following:

>> Weighing in at different times of the day

>> Eating right before stepping on the scale

>> Water weight fluctuations due to alcohol, menstrual cycles, and so on

To counteract these potential issues, try keeping tabs on the way your body looks and feels so you know exactly how well you are doing on your keto journey. Grab a tape measure and write down your waistline measurement once a week. Take photos in the same light, at the same time of day, and in the same location once a week. Pay attention to how your favorite clothes fit. Also take note of how much more energized you feel throughout the day as your body burns fat for energy.

Deciding Whether Keto Is Right for You

Keto can be adapted to fit anyone's needs — whether they're seeking to lose weight, reduce their risk of diabetes, or improve their energy levels. In this section, we give you a better idea of why keto may be right for you.

You want to lose weight and keep it that way

If you've tried other diets and felt discouraged because the weight either barely came off or didn't stay off, the keto diet is for you. Keto has been shown in dozens of studies to help people lose weight faster than low-fat, high-carb diets. Keto turns your body into a fat-burning machine — quite literally. When in ketosis, your body readily burns fat for energy, including stored fat! Even when being on a caloric deficit, keto dieters report that they don't really feel hungry like they do on other diets. This is a huge benefit that is not to be overlooked. On most diets, when you're hungry, your first instinct is to go to your fridge or pantry and devour the first tasty thing you see. You don't get that kind of hunger pang on keto, and it more often leads to your success and longevity with the diet.

You want to avoid becoming diabetic

Going keto or low-carb is the number one way of avoiding, controlling, and even reversing type 2 diabetes. Not eating carbohydrates means that you don't get blood glucose spikes, which in turn means that your insulin doesn't spike, and your cells don't become resistant to insulin. When your cells become insulin resistant, the pancreas tries to make more insulin to make the cells respond. Eventually, your pancreas can't keep up, and your blood sugar keeps rising or stays at a dangerously high level. Lowering insulin resistance is the primary method of reducing your chances of becoming diabetic. The keto diet can help reduce your risk of getting type 2 diabetes — a widespread problem that leads to heart disease and other major medical issues.

WARNING

Please be cautious if you have type 2 diabetes. Research is showing that the keto diet may help cure type 2 diabetes and get people off medications, but diabetes can be a severe medical condition that requires a doctor's care. It's best to have the support of a doctor if you've already been diagnosed with diabetes and take insulin regularly, because the keto diet will likely reduce the insulin dosage that is necessary. It can also lower your blood sugar levels too much if you're already taking certain medications.

You feel tired and sluggish most days

Most people who are on the keto diet for more than 3 weeks feel like they have more energy, consistent energy levels throughout the day, and better mental focus. Hunger pangs and that "hangry" feeling after not having a meal on schedule are a thing of the past. Getting sleepy after lunch just doesn't happen on keto. The reason these symptoms are practically universal is because normally on a high-carbohydrate diet, your body relies on higher blood sugar levels to then convert into energy with insulin. On keto, you get to break free of these symptoms because your blood sugar stays relatively stable through the day. Even if you skip a meal, your body switches to burning stored fat for energy. With keto, you're always energized and don't feel sluggish at the end of the day.

Knowing When to Stop

Most people are able to stay on the keto diet indefinitely. However, there are a few occasions when you should stop the diet and reassess your approach. Additionally, if you have type 1 diabetes, please speak with your doctor before trying keto or making any dietary changes.

Signs of danger

Here are a few signs to look for:

>> You feel tired all the time.

>> It's hard to sleep at night.

>> Your bathroom habits have ceased.

>> You feel weak or notice muscle loss.

>> You experience hair loss or rashes on your skin.

If you have any of these issues while on the keto diet, it may benefit you to speak with your doctor or take a pause to assess what is going wrong. Take stock of what you are eating and drinking and what your diet may be missing.

When you've achieved your goals

Keto is perfectly safe long-term, and there's no need to stop being in ketosis if that's not what you want. If you feel great on keto and don't want to quit, simply don't!

Although weight loss is achievable on any diet by being on a caloric deficit, keto has been proven to be the most effective diet in terms of speed and overall health indicators. If you've hit your ideal weight, you can increase your caloric intake by eating more fat and protein. Now you can enjoy more food with the same benefits.

You may choose to start eating more carbs again, and that's totally fine. However, be prepared because once you start eating more carbs, the energy highs and lows of the day come right back, along with sugar cravings. Suddenly, you're back to fighting with your willpower, exactly what you were able to eliminate with keto. Eating more complex carbs, lower on the glycemic index, is the best way to reintegrate and reduce blood-sugar spikes. The *glycemic index* is the food rating system with a scale of 1 to 100 that estimates how much a food will affect your blood-sugar levels. You'll gain a more in-depth understanding about the glycemic index in Chapter 3.

You may want to start building muscle while maintaining ketosis. If that's the case, increasing your protein calorie ratio to 30 or 35 percent and reducing your fat calorie ratio to 60 percent is the best way to do this. This is the basis of the high-protein keto diet you read about earlier in this chapter.

Additionally, when you work out, you'll be able to increase your total daily net carbs to around 50 grams because your body immediately burns the additional carbs, allowing you to stay in ketosis. Adding muscle mass is great for your health and makes it harder to regain fat.

You can also try experimenting with intermittent fasting. Basically, you get a specific window during the day to have your meals, but you get a lot more freedom. For example, you can try a time-restricted fast like 16 hours off food, 8 hours on. That translates to not eating 16 hours a day (sleep included) and eating during an 8-hour window. If you eat for the first time at 12 p.m., then you can eat up until 8 p.m. Reducing the eating window naturally limits the amount of food you can eat, so instead of weighing or measuring food to restrict your portions, you simply follow the clock.

The best part is you can combine intermittent fasting with any diet to reap the benefits. For more information on intermittent fasting, see Chapter 7.

Living a sustainable life on keto

Once you've achieved your weight loss goals, you can stop eating at a deficit by increasing your caloric intake to maintain your weight and essentially go on cruise control. As long-time keto dieters, we achieved our personal goals after about one year of being on keto. After that, we continued the keto lifestyle for more than 7 years and are still going. In our case, we stick to it because we feel great every day, have high energy levels, feel sharp and focused, and our annual physicals always come back with great results.

The keto diet became a lifestyle for us, and it can become a lifestyle for you too. Although doing it for the shorter-term can help you reap some of the benefits, the simple truth is it is very easy to fall back into old habits and reverse your progress. The bigger benefits come with sticking to it long-term. You may even find that by the time you reach your goals, you don't want to go back to eating carbs.

Chapter **2**

Considering Keto's Numerous Health Benefits

The keto diet is not only an amazing, delicious way to eat, but it has also been shown to improve your overall health. By eating high-quality, nutritious foods, you fuel your body with clean energy. This allows your body to be efficient, strong, and even resistant to many types of disease.

Switching to a low-carb, high-fat diet may seem overwhelming at first, especially if you're a bit rusty on topics like macros and metabolism. No need to worry! We guide you through the basics, which can help you breeze through many of the questions and misunderstandings that you may encounter from curious friends and family on your keto journey.

In this chapter, you discover the many benefits of keto — but get ready, it's not a short list! We also dive into the common misconception that fat is bad and makes you fat and how life without the real culprits — sugar and processed foods — can be so much sweeter.

Realizing All That Keto Has to Offer

The keto diet is not just a fad. It is a scientifically proven way to live a healthier life. Doctors have been aware of the benefits of ketosis since the early 1920s when they discovered ketones' ability to heal the body of a debilitating condition like *refractory epilepsy*, a form of epilepsy with which medicines don't work well, or at all, to control the seizures. Since then, there have been many more studies on the keto diet's benefits and discoveries that followed. When you recognize these benefits, you'll probably be as eager as we were to hop on the keto diet bandwagon.

Weight loss

We want to start out by clearing up a common misconception about fats. Eating fat does not make you fat. Fats can make you healthier! In fact, sugar and eating too many calories are the true causes of weight gain and poor health.

"Fat makes you fat" is a gimmick used by mega-corporations that fueled the high-sugar, low-fat diet craze of the 1980s and 1990s, which only managed to make many of us fatter, sicker, and addicted to sugar. Unfortunately, the number of people who struggle with obesity has doubled since that era.

When you go into ketosis, your body becomes a fat-burning machine. The fats you consume are immediately used by your body as energy. The more fats you have in your system, the more energy you have! Research has shown that people on a ketogenic diet increase their resting metabolism as well. This means your body is constantly working to break down the fatty acids in your system, giving you tons of energy and helping to jump-start your weight loss.

Not only does the keto diet help you lose weight by boosting energy levels, burning fats, and improving your metabolism, it also helps you shed pounds by decreasing cravings. It's natural to crave fatty foods when on a diet. Luckily, with keto, those foods are okay to eat! When you can satisfy your cravings and eat the high-fat foods you want, you're much happier and more likely to stick to your diet. Lose weight and eat delicious, fatty foods? It almost sounds too good to be true!

To take it a step further, consider the appetite hormone called *ghrelin*. Ghrelin is a hormone in your body that tells you when you are hungry. Research has shown that ghrelin levels rise when you reduce calories. Therefore, you always feel hungry on certain low-calorie diets. The high ghrelin levels are telling you to eat, eat, eat! However, when in ketosis, ghrelin levels fall drastically. Your body won't be telling you it's hungry even when you are losing weight.

When the body feeds off fats, it utilizes all the consumed fats as fuel and then more easily transitions over to using stored fats. You feel full and satisfied longer as your body is constantly feeding (and it's feeding off the fat you *want* to lose). This makes keto an easier diet to maintain and stick with.

REMEMBER

The ketogenic diet is a natural way to boost your metabolism and turn your body into a fat-burning machine. No starvation diet tricks or harmful chemicals are needed! Just your body's natural, already built-in metabolic process, which helps you achieve long-term weight loss.

Improved body composition

As we use our fat stores, we can whittle our waists, leading to improved cardio-vascular fitness. Belly fat is strongly associated with heart disease, high blood pressure, and diabetes. As we age, most of us lose muscle and gain fat naturally. Ketosis slows down this process. By switching to fat being the primary fuel source while providing enough protein through our diet, you maintain lean muscle mass because it's not used as a source of energy nearly as much as it is when you're on a high-carbohydrate diet.

Studies have shown that a keto diet versus a high-carb diet, when combined with exercise, have quite different results regarding total body fat and belly fat loss. In two studies, participants maintained the same strength-based routines. The ones on a keto diet lost more body fat and belly fat than those who ate a typical carbohydrate-rich diet (55 percent of their calories from carbohydrates, 25 percent from fat, and 20 percent from protein).

Increased energy

You may have heard a common misperception: that ketosis tricks your body into believing that it's starving. Although you do enter ketosis when you're starving, being in ketosis from eating fats and very few carbs does not mean you're starving. And being in ketosis is where the similarities end. Most importantly, you aren't hypoglycemic while on a keto diet. This means you won't have dangerously low levels of blood sugar that can leave you feeling lethargic, weak, dizzy, and "hangry." Many people we've come across, including physicians who aren't familiar with the diet, worry that ketosis will lead to a permanent state of exhaustion and lethargy or a dangerous drop in blood sugar. This simply isn't true — your blood glucose levels will be in the low end of the normal range but will always be stable due to a process called *gluconeogenesis*. Gluconeogenesis is a metabolic pathway that results in the generation of glucose from the breakdown of lipids (fats).

Compared to other diets, the keto diet is more likely to improve your energy levels. In a study looking at older individuals with type 2 diabetes who successfully followed a keto diet for over two years, researchers noticed an overall improvement in their quality of life compared to those who followed a low-fat, high-carb diet. Those in the keto group

>> Were better equipped to complete daily activities and chores

>> Experienced increased energy levels

>> Minimized routine body aches and pains

Overall, compared to a low-fat diet, multiple studies have proven that people feel better on a keto diet.

REMEMBER

On the keto diet, your glucose levels remain in a healthy range so you aren't risking the dangerous roller coaster of blood glucose and insulin spikes that can leave you lethargic, irritable, and just plain unhappy. Keto gets it right by keeping both your brain and your muscles efficient and energetic.

Improved mental focus

Ketosis is a natural way to gain more focus and mental clarity. Ketones stimulate *neurotrophins*, proteins that increase the development of brain cells and neurons. The ketones improve the neurons' resistance to stress and help with synaptic connections in the brain. This helps with memory and with the brain's ability to learn.

A few studies have shown that people on a keto diet are able to process information faster, learning new facts and retaining those facts more effectively. There is also lots of new excitement over the discovery that links the keto diet to treating neurodegenerative diseases, which are typically caused by metabolic inefficiency in the brain.

The keto diet is currently being used to help those with Alzheimer's disease and has been wildly successful. Patients have seen great improvements in memory, both short- and long-term.

REMEMBER

Ketones are a fantastic source of fuel for your body. A keto diet can help you focus, retain information, and even reverse neurodegenerative diseases.

Better sleep

We all need a good night's sleep to feel good, function properly, and have the energy we need to get through the day. Without rest, our brains have a hard time learning and retaining new information. Luckily, ketosis not only helps you fall asleep, but it may also help you have better-quality sleep.

The keto diet has been shown to increase the total amount of rapid eye movement (REM) sleep, which is a deep sleep state. Participants in a study who were on a keto diet needed fewer naps and maintained longer stretches of REM. The specifics of how ketones affect sleep are not yet fully understood, but the fact is, keto helps improve sleep.

REMEMBER

Your body may go through a short period of adjustment before you reach REM sleep. Some people may experience sleep problems when they first start the keto diet. Initially, the huge reduction in carb intake can cause changes to sleep patterns in a negative way. However, once your body adjusts, you will then transition into the deep, restful sleep you are looking for!

Stabilized blood sugar

About one-third of Americans are pre-diabetic and may not even know it. Diabetes and blood sugar issues are a huge problem but one that a keto diet can help. Ketosis is a state of perfect glucose control. Your glucose levels are never too high or too low but stable in a safe, healthy range.

Many people think that complex carbs are healthier than pure, refined sugar. However, once you eat those carbs, your body turns those carbs into glucose, although over a longer period. That glucose increases your blood-sugar levels and can increase your insulin resistance. So, even though you aren't eating pure sugar, you're still giving your body a huge dose of glucose.

Keto cuts back on drastic spikes in blood sugar. Without a huge dose of carbs at every meal, your blood sugar remains more stable and constant. This is much easier for your system to handle and doesn't cause nearly as much stress on your body.

Research has shown that people with type 2 diabetes do wonderfully on a low-carb diet like keto. A ketogenic diet can even help eliminate the need for diabetic medication since blood-sugar levels and insulin levels become relatively stable when eating a keto diet.

Many doctors recommend trying a ketogenic diet for those with type 2 diabetes. It can be wildly successful and can even eliminate the need for insulin or other blood-sugar controlling medications.

WARNING

Please consult with your doctor before starting keto if you're already diagnosed with diabetes and take insulin regularly. The keto diet is likely to reduce the insulin dosage that you're required to take. It may also lower your blood-glucose levels too much if you're already taking certain medications.

Healthier cholesterol levels

When you think of cholesterol, you may automatically think that it is bad. But cholesterol is a vital part of your cell membranes. There are four primary categories of cholesterol:

>> **Total cholesterol:** The total amount of cholesterol in your blood. This number on a lab report adds up all the categories of the following bullets and presents them as a single number.

>> **Low-density lipoprotein (LDL):** Often referred to as "bad" cholesterol. LDL is commonly associated with conditions like diabetes, strokes, and heart attacks.

>> **High-density lipoprotein (HDL):** Often referred to as "good" cholesterol. High levels of HDL are just the opposite of LDL; they tend to protect against diabetes, strokes, and heart attacks.

>> **Triglycerides:** Fats that are freely floating in your blood. These levels should rise when you eat a fatty meal but should go down to normal when you're fasting.

Low-carb diets, especially keto, help lower your total cholesterol levels (primarily made up of LDL) and triglycerides, while raising HDL. Keto also improves the HDL to total cholesterol ratio, another vital marker of heart health.

Another way the keto diet improves your health is by blocking an enzyme in your body called *HMG-CoA reductase*. This enzyme stimulates your liver, making more unhealthy cholesterol enter your blood stream. A low-carb diet prevents this enzyme from being produced which, in turn, inhibits the liver from producing too much cholesterol. When on a keto diet, many people find they don't need traditional cholesterol medicines, like statins, to control cholesterol levels — the diet does it naturally!

REMEMBER

In the long run, your diet affects your body more than anything else. Eating a nutritious keto diet complete with whole foods and high-quality ingredients helps you maintain healthy cholesterol levels and overall health.

Lower blood pressure

Another huge benefit of the keto diet is that the *amino acids* (protein building blocks) that are involved in ketosis are often blood-pressure-lowering proteins as opposed to acidifying amino acids, which are found in other metabolic states, (like glycolysis, which is the metabolic state you're in when you are eating a high-carb diet).

On average, Americans eat too much salt; we need only about 500 milligrams per day, and the average American gets more than 3,000 milligrams. For reference, 1 teaspoon of table salt is equal to 2,300 milligrams.

Salt is typically linked to higher blood pressure, so many people abstain from eating salt as a tool to control blood pressure. Being in ketosis can also actually lower the amount of salt your body retains. Additionally, the keto diet naturally eliminates many processed high-carb foods that are high in salt, so you naturally consume less salt. That fact, combined with the amino acids from ketosis that lower blood pressure, mean the keto diet is perfect for anyone watching their blood pressure levels. In fact, many people on keto can indulge in adding more salt to their meals because they're much more likely to be closer to or lower than the recommended salt levels than the average American.

The foods in the keto diet are often high in nutrients like potassium, iron, zinc, and antioxidants. Eating whole, high-quality foods also has a positive effect on blood pressure. Just the act of eliminating processed foods and unhealthy carbs from your diet has a positive effect immediately. By switching to a keto diet, you don't have to think as much about avoiding blood pressure–increasing foods because it happens naturally.

Reduced acne

Many studies have shown that people who eat more carbs and high glycemic foods have higher levels of insulin, which can lead to increased inflammation of skin cells. Inflamed skin means clogged pores and acne. Reducing your intake of these carb-loaded foods helps your skin heal, preventing future acne and even helping improve the appearance of acne scars.

Dermatologists are catching on to keto and are seeing success after switching their patients to a low-carb eating style. Many studies of people with moderate or severe acne have shown that sticking to a low-carb or keto diet is associated with a decrease in severity of acne and acne scars.

If you are struggling with acne and topical products aren't working, it may be time to consider your diet as the cause of your skin issues. It may just be all those excess carbohydrates.

Fewer PCOS symptoms

If you suffer from polycystic ovarian syndrome (PCOS), you'll be pleased to know that the keto diet has been proven to help decrease its effects and often effectively eliminate it entirely.

The traditional treatment route for PCOS is to basically treat the symptom(s). If a patient has irregular periods, birth control pills are prescribed to regulate the periods. If a patient has infertility, they are given fertility treatments, although they are often unsuccessful due to other PCOS complications.

Just like type 2 diabetes, insulin resistance plays a major role in developing PCOS. By improving insulin resistance through the keto diet, PCOS symptoms are often greatly improved. In one study, about a third of the participants had their periods return after not having had one for several years, and in the same study, a third of the participants became pregnant after many years of failure due to PCOS.

Because the keto diet helps with insulin resistance, weight loss, inflammation, and many other issues that often cause PCOS, it effectively acts as an all-in-one treatment for PCOS.

If you're starting the keto diet to try to manage your PCOS, be sure to work with your healthcare provider so they can monitor your progress closely.

Less inflammation

Inflammation is another way to say "immune activity." It's a combination of white blood cells, cytokines, platelets, and other immune items, which are released or sent by the body in response to an injury, infection, or illness.

When you have a cut, your body works to heal it quickly by clotting blood to stop the bleeding and form a scab, sending white blood cells to kill any bacteria in the area and then letting the skin slowly regenerate in that area. That's called *acute inflammation*, which is caused in response to a specific injury with a specific purpose.

Chronic inflammation is when your body constantly has a low-grade immune response with no useful purpose. It's an unnecessary inflammation that causes damage and increases the risk for a whole host of diseases like heart disease, diabetes, and Alzheimer's. A lot of things drive chronic inflammation, but the bigger ones are high-carb diets, sleep deprivation, cigarette smoking, and aging.

Ketones are anti-inflammatory signaling molecules. Studies have shown that keto diets decrease a variety of inflammation-associated illnesses like type 2 diabetes and Alzheimer's.

Here are a few keto approved foods that are also anti-inflammatory:

>> Avocado oil

>> Nuts and seeds

>> Coconut oil

>> Salmon

>> Eggs

>> Leafy greens

Following are some of the major inflammatory foods that you should *avoid*:

>> Table sugar and refined sugar like high-fructose corn syrup

>> Vegetable oils like soybean, corn, sunflower, and grapeseed oil

>> Artificial trans fats like stick margarine, commercial baked goods, and microwave popcorn

The keto diet alone helps you reduce inflammation, but these foods take it a step further, filling you with anti-inflammatory nutrients like omega-3 fatty acids and beneficial vitamins.

Disease prevention

It is incredible how the keto diet works with your body, combating diseases simply through the elimination of carbs. So many health issues are exacerbated by too many carbs, and switching to a fat-based diet improves conditions without even targeting them. Here, we take a look at a few conditions that the keto diet helps, so you may be even more excited to begin on your keto journey.

Epilepsy

The keto diet was first created to treat epilepsy. In the 1920s, doctors found that children with epilepsy showed great improvement when fasting. Because long-term fasting was not an option, doctors turned to low-carb diets to put the body into ketosis, which reduced a huge percentage of the seizures the children were having.

Doctors found that the ketogenic diet reduces the amount of *glutamate* in the brain, a chemical that nerve cells use to send signals to other cells. When there is too much of this neurotransmitter in the brain, nerve cells can fire too frequently, which results in a seizure. Being able to limit and reduce the amount of glutamate in a natural way via diet is incredible.

To this day, many hospitals and programs like Johns Hopkins', still use a strict keto diet to treat patients with epilepsy. With the advances in anti-seizure medications, keto is used a little less in the current day, but it is still a method some doctors try. It is even approved for those with rare forms of seizures that don't respond to anti-seizure medications.

Diabetes and other metabolic disorders

Did you know that one in ten people around the world suffer from diabetes? It is a terrible metabolic syndrome that is associated with insulin resistance, abnormal cholesterol levels, and high blood pressure. The keto diet can not only treat but also possibly reverse type 2 diabetes and metabolic syndrome.

Eating too many carbs increases glucose levels and leads to insulin insufficiency. When people with diabetes switch to a keto diet, their blood glucose levels drastically improve. Those who can stick with the keto diet may reverse their diabetes completely and be able to stop medication.

Treating diabetes with keto is an idea that has been around since the 1970s. Keep in mind that the keto diet is a great way to treat type 2 diabetes, *not* type 1. Type 2 diabetes is typically lifestyle related and develops over time. The keto diet can help reverse type 2 diabetes by helping the body lower glucose levels consistently and reduce insulin resistance. It is tried-and-true and can help almost anyone with type 2 diabetes.

Fibromyalgia

Fibromyalgia is a chronic condition that causes ongoing, severe pain. Millions of people around the world suffer from fibromyalgia, but it is also a catch-all term that doctors use when they aren't sure how to treat chronic pain. Pain medications just mask the problem further.

Researchers believe that one of the underlying causes of fibromyalgia is inflammation. Many people with fibromyalgia have sugar and hormone imbalances, over-excited pain sensors, free radicals, and poor liver function. All these conditions wreak havoc on the body, causing neurons to fire repeatedly, eventually leading to damage. Poor liver health, which blocks your body's ability to get rid of toxins or inflammatory particles (like free radicals), further damages our pain nerves and muscles, causing us to feel pain with no trigger.

By changing your diet and resisting harmful carbs and sugary foods, you can address the inflammatory cause of fibromyalgia pain. The keto diet can help to not only decrease inflammation but also decrease your response to the sensation of pain.

Cardiovascular disease

Heart disease is the leading cause of death in the world. In fact, one in every four deaths in the United States is due to heart disease. It is a major problem that needs a solution. But many people are afraid to turn to a high-fat diet when cardiovascular disease is such a major issue, and they've been told their whole lives that fat is bad.

High-fat diets are often associated with *atherosclerosis*, a type of heart disease where the arterial walls are damaged by free radicals in the blood, causing plaque to build up and restrict blood flow in arteries. Inflammation plays a big part in this process as well. Plaque can only build up if you have a damaged arterial wall, and the primary cause of damage is typically inflammation. If you can decrease inflammation, you will reduce the risk of plaque buildup.

Remember when we talked about the keto diet controlling cholesterol? This all comes into play here! The keto diet may be high in fats, but it is the king of good fats and the good types of cholesterol.

The keto diet does the following things, all of which are fantastic for your heart health:

» Helps you reach a healthy weight, which is easier on your heart and all major organs

» Improves blood-sugar levels

» Is anti-inflammatory, which helps keep your arteries undamaged and open for blood to easily flow through

» Helps blood cholesterol levels by balancing LDL and HDL

All these benefits help decrease the risk of strokes and heart attacks. People who eat healthy, low-carb, whole foods have a much lower risk of cardiovascular disease. It is incredible to think that a simple dietary change may help reduce the amount of cardiovascular disease in the world.

UNDERSTANDING THE AMAZING MEDICAL ORIGINS OF KETO

The keto diet was created in the 1920s to treat epilepsy. It was used as a therapeutic, natural way to reduce seizures. Patients who were in ketosis experienced far fewer epileptic episodes; some even experienced no seizures at all! The discovery was truly incredible.

Dr. Robert Atkins then wrote about the keto diet (he called it the low-carb diet, but effectively it was the same thing) in 1972 in his book: *Dr. Atkins' Diet Revolution: The High Calorie Way to Stay Thin Forever*. The Atkins diet gained popularity in the early 1990s and within a few years, one in eleven North American adults claimed to be on a low-carb diet. The Atkins diet starts out as ultra-low carb (keto) but then slowly adds carbs back to the diet so it's not a true keto diet over the long term.

Fortunately, around 2005, extensive research on low-carb diets began due to the popularity of the Atkins diet, and we're continuing to find out more about the benefits of long-term ketosis today.

Chapter **3**

Transforming Your Kitchen into a Keto Kitchen

Are you ready to get rid of all those unhealthy carbs that are lurking in your pantry? We are ready to help you! Before you start a keto diet, you need to take a hard look in your fridge, pantry, and that snack drawer you have in your office and clear out any carb-heavy foods. But don't worry! We will help you replace them with whole-food, keto items that taste even better and will keep you satisfied and feeling full for hours.

Following the keto diet is going to transform your body, but this also means transforming your kitchen. Your mind and your pantry both need to be reset when it comes to food and eating. This chapter tells you all about how to do that in a practical and efficient way.

REMEMBER

Keep in mind that you will not be sacrificing flavor when you go keto. One of the trademarks of the keto diet is that you get to enjoy delicious, mouth-watering foods.

Out with the Old

Sadly, most of us have a pantry filled with carb-packed foods. Bread, rice, flour, and pasta are staple ingredients in many households. These may have been your go-to ingredients in the past, but they won't work as part of a keto diet. But don't worry! We are here to help you get rid of these foods and replace them with keto-friendly foods that have a whole lot more nutritional value.

Getting rid of hidden sugars in your kitchen

Sugar is one of the biggest culprits when it comes to weight gain. Sugar drives your insulin levels up and causes your body to store extra fat. When you consume a lot of sugar, you are fighting an uphill battle when it comes to achieving a healthy weight. Cutting these excess sugars is the first step toward shedding pounds and getting healthy.

When you think of sugar, you probably automatically think of white granulated sugar. But what about alternative sugars? Honey, coconut sugar, and fruit sweeteners, like dates, are all still sugars. Yes, they have antioxidants and fiber, but despite their possible benefits, they are still, at the core, sugar. When you start your keto journey, all sugar needs to go.

Here are the sugars that you need to get rid of and remove from your pantry:

>> **Brown, white, or turbinado sugar:** All of these are made from sugar cane and have very high calorie and carb content. Avoid all white, brown, and even the less processed turbinado sugar.

>> **Coconut sugar:** Coconut sugar is said to be "healthier" than granulated white sugar because it has a lower glycemic index. (For more information on the glycemic index, see the sidebar later in this chapter.) It also has traces of fiber and some other nutrients. But the bottom line is that it is still sugar. It still causes your blood sugar to spike. Coconut sugar is not part of the keto diet.

>> **Sucanat:** Sucanat is a type of sugar cane sweetener that is minimally processed. It is also known as muscovado, jaggery, and panela. Even though it is not heavily processed, it is still sugar. It kicks you out of ketosis and raises your blood sugar levels almost instantly.

>> **Honey:** Honey does have some benefits such as antioxidant properties and anti-inflammatory effects. But the bottom line is that it is still sugar. Honey has more calories than sugar and causes your blood sugar to rise just like every other sugar. It's not okay on the keto diet.

>> **Molasses:** Molasses is a less processed product of sugar cane, but it is still 75 percent sugar (the remaining part being water and trace minerals). You probably guessed that it is not okay for the keto diet. Don't worry though — you get far more minerals from delicious keto foods.

>> **Agave:** Agave is another natural sweetener that is made primarily of fructose. High levels of fructose can cause liver damage and increase weight gain. It may be worse for you than white sugar. Skip anything that uses agave as a sweetener.

>> **Dates:** Dates are often seen as a better-for-you sugar. Dates are made from 80 percent sugar, with three dates containing about 50 grams of sugar. It is very easy to fall out of ketosis by using dates as a sweetener. Dates are a great example of a food that may be natural or organic but still needs to be avoided on the keto diet.

>> **Syrups:** Maple syrup, corn syrup, and rice syrup are all essentially sugary water.

If you have bottles or bags of these sugary ingredients, be sure to get rid of them before starting a keto diet. You should also be sure to discard anything that may contain any of these sugars. Cookies, chips, and even crackers may need to go. Once again, we promise to tell you how to replace everything with fantastic keto foods.

TIP

Plan a day to go through your pantry, fridge, and entire kitchen. You want to check nutrition labels and ingredient lists to see what is inside every food you have. Make piles of keto foods and non-keto foods. You will be very surprised by how many processed foods have hidden sugars. Reading all the labels will give you a firm grasp on how prevalent sugar is in our Western diet.

REMEMBER

Most ingredient labels don't simply list "sugar." You may have to dive deeper and do a little detective work to assess whether a food has sugar or not.

Here are a few alternate names for sugar that you should memorize:

>> Maltodextrin

>> Cane sugar

>> Dextrose

>> Fruit juice concentrate

>> Sucrose

>> High-fructose corn syrup

>> Glucose

WARNING

Artificial sugars and no-calorie sweeteners can be great; however, you should always be cautious when using them. They may still spike your blood-sugar levels. Anytime you eat something that is sweet, the receptors on your tongue may tell your body to prepare for carbs. This can automatically raise your blood sugar as your body prepares for those carbs and starts creating insulin. Some studies show that certain sweeteners, like sucralose, can still spike insulin even though they do not contain calories or carbs. This can lead to weight gain, diabetes, or heart disease as a result of the high insulin levels. Remember that the goal with keto is to avoid increases in blood-sugar levels and insulin spikes. Here are a few artificial sweeteners you may want to avoid:

>> Sucralose (Splenda)

>> Acesulfame potassium (Ace-K, Sunett)

>> Aspartame (NutraSweet)

>> Saccharin (Sweet'n Low)

>> Mixed sweeteners (Equal)

Goodbye to flours, grains, and starchy veggies

We talked a little bit about "hidden carbs," which are the carbs and sugars you may not even know are there. Simple sugars, like the ones we talk about in the preceding section, are easy to identify. Complex carbs can be trickier.

You probably know that white flour is a carb. But what about whole wheat and whole grains? They are carbs as well. While whole grains may contain some nutrients, they are still not keto friendly. They increase your blood-sugar levels and kick you out of ketosis quite quickly. Whether they are "healthy" or not, your body ultimately sees whole grains as a sugar and treats them that way. You can easily get the same nutrients from other, keto-safe foods so there is no need for whole grains in your diet.

Here is a quick look at the grains and flours that you want to ditch:

>> Whole wheat and white flours

>> Couscous

>> All wheat pasta

>> White rice, brown rice, and wild rice

- » Millet
- » Barley
- » Quinoa
- » Oats
- » Amaranth
- » Teff
- » Sorghum

REMEMBER

"Ancient grains" are often touted as being very healthy, but they are still, essentially, carbs. All the nutrition in ancient grains can easily be found elsewhere in keto-safe foods.

One of the trickiest foods to eliminate may just be starchy veggies. You may not realize how many carbs are in some veggies since we often just look at a vegetable and automatically think it is "healthy." However, many vegetables are packed with carbs that may harm your state of ketosis.

Here are the starchy vegetables you want to avoid:

- » Root vegetables and tubers (potatoes, carrots, squash)
- » Beans, green peas, and lentils
- » Corn and cornmeal
- » Plantains
- » Pumpkin

Even when cooked, many of these foods are considered high glycemic and increase your insulin levels. Ditch all these starchy veggies and stick to the nutritious vegetables that won't boost your blood sugar.

Tossing high-glycemic fruits

Many fruits do not work on the keto diet. They are far too high in sugars and raise your blood glucose significantly. There are quite a few fruits that you can enjoy on the keto diet without a negative impact. So, don't worry if you're a fruit lover, you still get to eat some very tasty fruits.

GLYCEMIC INDEX

The glycemic index (GI) is a system that rates foods on a scale of 1 to 100 based on their effect on blood-sugar levels. Foods that have a higher glycemic value spike blood sugar more and faster. High GI foods should be completely avoided on the keto diet.

Watermelon, for example, has a GI of 72, which means eating a slice will boost your blood sugar way up, make your body produce extra insulin, and send you out of ketosis. Blueberries, on the other hand, have a GI of only 53. This is why a keto dieter can enjoy a handful of blueberries but not a few slices of watermelon.

The glycemic index is a good tool to help you decide which foods are okay on a keto diet. It can be beneficial to see hard numbers like this, especially when you first start assessing foods for their keto-compatibility.

Here are a few high-glycemic fruits that you should avoid when on the keto diet:

>> Apples

>> Bananas

>> Mangoes

>> Oranges

>> Kiwis

>> Pineapples

Purging all processed foods

Almost all processed foods have to go. This can be hard on your kitchen and pantry, but the truth is that most of those processed foods you have in your home are not nutritious at all. Packaged foods are designed to last a long time on the shelf. They have preservatives and chemicals added to the food to accomplish this goal. These additives can damage your body in the long run.

Many processed foods also have sugars and artificial sweeteners added in. Your brain is designed to seek out sweet foods, so companies add sweetness to their food to attract you and make you like their product. Check the nutrition labels on any packaged foods you want to buy and, if you see one of these ingredients on the label, it's most likely off limits.

- » High-fructose corn syrup
- » Soybean, palm, corn, or canola oil
- » Hydrogenated oils
- » Artificial flavors
- » Monosodium glutamate

TIP

When grocery shopping, try to stick to the "outer ring" of the store where all the fresh foods are. Produce, meat, and refrigerated foods are always on the outer walls of the store, and this is where you find the fresh, natural foods. About 90 percent of your foods should come from the outer ring.

Working with multiple diets in the same kitchen

If you are in a mixed household where some people are following keto and others are not, it may get a little more complicated in your kitchen. You can't exactly throw away your roommate's bag of chips and cookies without causing issues. This can be very hard for those trying to live a keto lifestyle as temptation can be lurking in the pantry. We want to give you a few tips and tricks to help navigate the challenges of a shared kitchen.

- » Reorganize your drawers, pantry, and fridge to have a keto section and a non-keto section. Try labeling all your keto foods and setting them to one side so it is easy to see what you can eat and what you should avoid.

- » Try to make your keto meals first so you are not tempted by the cooking smells of non-keto foods. If you must prepare non-keto foods for your family or kids, eating your own keto dinner first may be a good idea. Then you will be full and happy while you prep other non-keto meals.

- » Serve keto foods to your family and friends. There are so many fantastic keto meals that everyone can enjoy. Even if you don't convince people to switch to a keto diet, they can still appreciate and enjoy a keto meal.

- » If you are doing intermittent fasting, try to line up your fasting schedule with your family's eating schedule. Match up the times you eat with the times you will be sitting down at the table together. This helps you avoid temptation during a fast.

REMEMBER

It can be tricky to cater to multiple diets from one kitchen, but it's not impossible. Know the foods that are okay on a keto diet and stick to them. Labeling foods that are keto approved can be a huge help. Try putting a big "K" on anything that is safe for you.

Tips for organizing cabinets

As we mention earlier, we love labels, especially when it comes to the keto diet. Adding labels to foods that are keto safe can be a huge help, especially when you are new to the keto lifestyle. Having the visual of a keto label allows you to quickly open your cabinet, see which foods are keto, and grab them easily. This is especially helpful if you still have non-keto foods in your home.

Cooking from Scratch Gives You an Advantage

Cooking keto foods from scratch is a fantastic way to ensure you eat tasty, healthy keto meals. You get a huge advantage when you choose your own recipe and prepare your own foods. Cooking gives you complete control over the ingredients you use, so you never need to worry whether or not a food is keto friendly.

We give you tons of incredible keto recipes in Parts 2–5 of this book that you can try. These recipes are a great place to start your keto journey. However, when you have already cleaned out your kitchen, ridding it of non-keto ingredients, you can also rest assured that the ingredients you have on hand are keto. We strongly recommend going through your pantry and following the previous tips to make your kitchen keto and *then* start cooking.

Caloric availability

Caloric availability is the number of calories your body can receive from a food. This is calculated by adding up all the components in a food, such as the carbohydrates, proteins, fats, and all the other nutrients. Food labels list the caloric number at the top of the food label so you know how many calories to expect to consume when eating that food.

But not all calories are the same. Your body may not absorb all the calories from certain foods, making them lower in calories than you may have thought. For example, a food that is high in protein and fiber is harder for the body to digest. Because your body pushes these foods out of your digestive tract faster, the calories in the foods are not always absorbed, which means you get all the pleasures of eating these foods but fewer calories.

Sugar and carbs, on the other hand, are very easy for the body to process. They have a much higher caloric availability and, in turn, cause weight gain. The keto diet, by nature, has low caloric availability. This is just another reason why the keto diet can help you lose weight!

TIP

The calories listed on a food nutrition label may not truly reflect how many calories your body absorbs. Foods that are high in fiber, for example, often provide fewer calories than their labels reflect.

When you start cooking your own keto meals, keep this in mind and try to add fiber to your diet. This helps to improve your digestive system and keep your body regular.

Customizing recipes based on food sensitivities, allergies, and preferences

Preparing your own foods is fantastic, especially because you can customize recipes to suit your personal nutritional needs. You can choose recipes that already fit into your dietary needs, or you can adjust recipes to make them perfect for you.

If a recipe contains a high-allergen food, you can often easily replace certain ingredients. For example, a recipe that contains peanut butter can be altered by using almond butter or nut-free sun butter in place of peanut butter at a 1:1 replacement amount. Another example is replacing heavy cream or half-and-half with coconut milk or almond milk.

Buying processed foods does not give you this flexibility. You are stuck eating what the food manufacturer gives you. This can be very hard for someone who is trying to go keto and has food sensitivities or allergies. While cooking and preparing foods may be more time consuming, keep in mind these great benefits. You are in complete control of what you eat and completely able to customize all your meals.

Meal prepping

Meal prepping or batch cooking is a great way to help you prepare days of keto meals with little effort. The idea is to create all your keto meals ahead of time, doing the bulk of the cooking and work in one day so the rest of your week is easier.

Set aside an hour or two one day and use this time to cook extra veggies, proteins, or side dishes. Package them up in individual containers and label them with the days of the week. On that day, you will be able to grab the prepped meal or side dish, warm it up in a few minutes if necessary, and eat! After just one day of cooking, you can take the rest of the week off.

Meal prep really helps you stay on the keto track as well. Since you are doing most of your cooking on one day, you can really focus on the ingredients you use, keeping them in line with your keto needs.

Meal prep also makes tracking calories and macros a lot easier. (See Chapter 5 for more on macros.) You can do the calculations for each prepped meal (breakfast, lunch, and dinner) and then apply it to the days you're eating that meal without having to recalculate each time.

REMEMBER

Home cooking and proper preparation help you on your keto journey. They give you total control of your foods and keep you actively invested in your diet routine. This helps you stick to your diet and understand keto fully.

Saving money

Preparing your own foods saves you money in the long run. Packaged foods cost much more than raw ingredients. You are paying for convenience, but those "convenient" foods aren't necessarily worth the money.

One way to be sure you get your money's worth on produce, meats, and other fresh ingredients is to be sure you use everything. Don't let that bag of spinach go bad in your fridge! Instead, do meal prep to ensure everything gets used and, in turn, eaten. Reducing waste helps you save money.

Stock up on keto ingredients that are on sale. Many veggies and proteins freeze well. If you see chicken thighs on sale, for example, buy extra and then freeze them. Anytime you need chicken, you will have it, and you will have locked in that discount price.

If you're trying to be healthier by purchasing organic foods, choosing organic animal products and animal byproducts is a must due to antibiotic feeding of animals that are not being organically farmed. However, for fruits and veggies, there is some leeway, especially for fruit and non-root vegetables. Splurge on organic when it comes to

>> All fruit, especially berries (strawberries, blueberries, raspberries, and so on)

>> Spinach

>> Celery

>> Tomatoes

>> Peppers

Although you won't be eating many fruits that aren't berries, you may have the occasional apple in a salad, like coleslaw, or have smaller portions of larger fruit to enjoy occasionally, while maintaining ketosis. So be sure to buy organic fruit regardless.

REMEMBER

Buying raw ingredients and preparing your keto foods in advance saves you a lot of time and money, as well as mental and physical effort throughout the week (less thinking about what to make, gathering ingredients, calculating macros, cooking, and so forth).

Chapter **4**

Choosing Keto-Appropriate Foods and Ingredients

After getting rid of all the non-keto-friendly foods from your pantry shelves and fridge, you may be wondering what you can eat when you're on a keto diet. It's finally time to go shopping. There are tons of amazing foods that you can enjoy. By the end of this chapter, you will be a keto ingredient master.

Discovering How to Shop for Keto

It can be overwhelming to wrap your head around a whole new way to shop. There are plenty of keto ingredients you can use, but many staple foods you may have enjoyed in the past are now off your list. It can take a while to figure out how to shop and navigate away from the carb-heavy foods of your past.

Keep in mind the grocery store rule we talk about in Chapter 3: Stick to the "outer rim" of the grocery store. The foods against the outer walls tend to be fresh, natural foods. While they aren't all keto, you will find many, many keto items here. It's a good place to start.

Before you head to the grocery store, you should pick out a few keto recipes that you want to make. Having recipes in mind can help you make your grocery list and push you to only buy keto-friendly ingredients. There are apps that can help you generate grocery lists from keto recipes, making your shopping job even easier. The Total Keto Diet App, for example, not only has tons of delicious recipes for you to scroll through, but it can also create a shopping list for you. Could it be any easier than that? Keto shopping doesn't have to be hard.

The keto diet is a high-fat way of eating, so you want to be sure to incorporate lots of healthy fats into your diet and your shopping list. Fat is the primary source of fuel for your body on keto, and luckily for us, it makes foods taste incredible!

Stocking up on eggs

Eggs are an incredible source of nutrition. They have lots of healthy fats, beneficial protein, and healthy micronutrients. On the keto diet, you can eat the whole egg, including the yolk. No need to ask for just egg whites ever again!

Eggs are a good source of choline, a nutrient that is important to metabolism and brain health. They have anti-inflammatory minerals like zinc and selenium. Contrary to popular belief, eggs do not cause high blood-cholesterol levels, and studies have shown that eating eggs does not increase the risk of heart disease.

We especially love eggs because they can be eaten in a wide variety of ways. You can make hard-boiled eggs, fried eggs, or give a tasty frittata a try.

Try to buy local farm-raised eggs, if possible. These eggs are the healthiest and the tastiest. If you need to buy your eggs from a grocery store, we recommend spending the extra money on organic, pasture-raised eggs. They should have the highest amount of omega-3 fatty acids, vitamins, minerals, and healthy fats that you are looking for. Be sure to read the label on the egg carton. Egg manufacturers like to use quite a few terms to entice you to buy their eggs.

Here is a quick look at some of those terms and what they mean:

>> **Omega-3 enriched:** This means that the chickens were fed a diet high in omega-3 feed, typically flaxseed. Keep in mind that this term is not highly regulated. Egg manufacturers can label their eggs as "omega-3 enriched" without adhering to any investigation or standards.

>> **Vegetarian fed:** These chickens are usually fed a diet of corn and soy. This isn't the healthiest diet for a chicken. While it may sound nice that a chicken was fed only vegetarian feed, it doesn't really contain the most nutritious grains.

- **» Cage free:** Unfortunately, this term is quite misleading. Most cage-free chickens are not roaming a field, happy and free. Instead, they are packed into a room, allowed to roam only in a space full of several hundred chickens. Technically, there are no cages, but there also isn't much "roaming space."

- **» Farm-fresh or natural:** These terms have no specifications or regulations. Any eggs can be labeled "natural" since they are made naturally by a chicken. Don't be fooled into paying double the price for "farm-fresh" eggs. They likely are not from your local farm.

- **» Pasture-raised:** We always look for pasture-raised eggs because this is a term that has meaning. These chickens are allowed to come and go from the barn, allowing them to get real sunlight, forage for worms, and get some exercise. All these things contribute to making good, nutritious eggs!

- **» Free range or free roaming:** The standards for these terms are a little bit better than "cage free." The chickens are typically kept in large barns and have some freedom of movement. However, there are still no strict rules that regulate how much the chickens can move or the type of terrain they are in, factors that are important to egg development.

- **» Certified organic:** This label has some strict rules attached to it. Chickens must be antibiotic and pesticide free. They need an all-vegetarian diet and to have access to the outside. However, outdoor time and environment are not regulated and, as we mention earlier, a vegetarian diet may not be best for chickens. Yet with organic eggs, at least you know you're purchasing eggs that have some controls put on their creation.

In a nutshell, pasture-raised eggs are the best when you must buy eggs from the grocery store. Locally sourced eggs from a real farm are always the most nutritious. Buy your eggs wisely as they can be a wonderful, healthy addition to a keto diet.

REMEMBER

Choosing high-quality eggs is essential. The nutritional value of eggs can really vary based on the treatment of the chickens. Chickens who are raised outside in the sunshine lay eggs that are higher in vitamin D. Those who eat feed enriched with omega-3 fatty acids lay omega-3 rich eggs.

Opting for fattier cuts of meat and poultry

Now that you are on a keto diet, you get to enjoy all the luscious flavors of full-fat meats. Don't worry about having a few saturated fats in your diet. Saturated fat has been shown not to have a direct link to heart disease or stroke as some previously thought, especially when you're on a keto diet. So, add some of your favorite fatty meats back into your diet.

Here are our favorites:

- » Chicken thighs
- » Tenderloin
- » Porterhouse
- » Skirt steak
- » T-bone
- » Ribeye
- » Flap steak
- » New York strip
- » Pork or beef ribs

Try to buy healthy, minimally processed meats. Unprocessed meats are healthier and have less preservatives that can harm your system. Processed meats tend to contain higher amounts of salt and, of course, preservatives, that can increase the risk of heart disease. Stick to natural, pure meat rather than deli-style meats.

REMEMBER

Always opt for quality when you eat these meats. Just like we talk about the quality of eggs being affected by the environment, the quality of meat is also altered by how the animals are treated and raised. Look for grass-fed; antibiotic-free; and ideally, organic meat.

TIP

Don't be afraid to try new meats. Exploring new ways of eating is a big part of being on the keto diet. Wild meats like bison, duck, and pheasant are great options that you may have never tried before. Many of these animals are free-range and have high nutritional content. The quality and taste speak for themselves.

Fishing for fatty seafood

Perhaps you are a seafood person rather than a meat person. You're in luck! Seafood is a great source of fatty protein and omega-3s, and it's an excellent source of vitamin D. Vitamin D is not only important for bone health, but it also improves your immune system. It has even been shown to improve your mood. Vitamin D can be tough to get, especially if you live in a cold climate where going out in the sun isn't always possible. Wild-caught fish can help you get the vitamin D and minerals that you need. Farmed fish is still a great option, but always look for the wild fish in your local grocery store. Just as with eggs and meats, wild and natural are always best!

Here are a few of our favorite fatty fishes that you can easily add to your keto diet:

>> Salmon

>> Mackerel

>> Catfish

>> Trout

>> Anchovies

>> Sardines

REMEMBER

Some oily fish have been shown to have high amounts of mercury. Salmon and catfish are lower in mercury and very safe choices of fatty fish.

Going high fat in the dairy aisle

High-fat dairy is a very good option when on a keto diet. Dairy is high in calcium, which contributes to bone health. The fats in the dairy give you a good source of energy, which your body needs when in ketosis.

Skip the low-fat or skim products and go right for the tasty, creamier options.

Lactose is the main sugar found in milk, and it adds to your carb count. However, full-fat dairy has lower levels of lactose than low-fat dairy. Just another reason why you should go with the extra fat! A little bit of cow's milk here and there is okay on keto, but it's better to switch to half-and-half or heavy cream in your coffee.

Cheese, on the other hand, has most of the lactose completely removed. Hard, aged cheeses have less lactose than soft cheese, so you should try to stick to the hard cheeses when following a keto diet.

You can eat a lot of dairy, and your body will still stay in ketosis.

Here are a few of our favorite keto-approved dairy options:

>> Cheddar cheese

>> Parmesan cheese

>> Heavy cream

>> Full-fat yogurt

>> Butter

>> Swiss cheese

Feel free to use a lot of butter for cooking and baking keto foods. You can use salted or unsalted butter; both are completely keto safe. Look for grass-fed butter, which has much more nutritional value and is healthier overall.

REMEMBER

Dairy does still have lactose, and lactose is a carb. Limit the amount of milk you drink and try to stick to hard cheeses, which have less lactose. Always choose full-fat dairy, which is less processed, more nutritious, and has less natural lactose.

Picking the best cooking oils

When you start a keto diet, fat becomes the most important macronutrient in your diet. When you are following a diet that focuses on fats, you can fry, sauté, and baste foods in fats as much as you'd like to. Since you will be using a lot of oil for cooking, you should make sure you know all about the type of oil you choose.

Low-quality oils are often processed with chemicals, which remove any nutrients the oil used to have. Look for oils that are minimally processed to ensure you get all the benefits possible from the fats.

High-quality oils are often labeled with terms such as "virgin" or "expeller pressed." Knowing what these terms mean can help you decide which type of oil to buy:

>> **Virgin and extra virgin:** The oil is pressed at a lower heat than expeller-pressed oils. Extra-virgin oil is pressed only once, getting the purest, smoothest oil possible. Virgin oil can be pressed more than once but still utilizes the low heat or cold-pressed methods, making it unprocessed and pure.

>> **Expeller pressed:** This term implies that the seeds were pressed at high heats and with high pressure.

>> **Refined oil:** Refined oil is made using chemicals, which extract the fats from the seeds in a quick and very cheap way. These oils are not very nutritious and often very cheap.

Virgin and extra-virgin oils have been shown to have a higher level of nutrients such as antioxidants and minerals. Virgin oil even has a better taste and smell, which adds to the overall flavor of your cooking. Here are a few oils that we recommend using within your keto diet:

>> **Virgin coconut oil:** Coconut oil has over 90 perfect fat, which makes it fantastic for keto cooking. It has a high smoke point so you can bake or even roast foods using coconut oil. Studies have shown that people who eat high amounts of coconut oil have higher levels of "good" cholesterol.

>> **Extra-virgin olive oil:** Olive oil comes from olives, which are full of beneficial nutrients. People who cook with olive oil on a regular basis have been shown to have stable blood pressure and a lower risk for cardiovascular disease. Extra-virgin olive oil is also anti-inflammatory and a known antioxidant. Try frying and baking with olive oil or just use it to make a quick salad dressing.

>> **Avocado oil:** Avocado oil is high in monounsaturated fats and very low in polyunsaturated fats. It's also rich in vitamins A, B1, B2, D, and E. Avocado oil has the highest smoke points of all the oils, around 500°F, which makes it ideal for all frying and baking purposes. It also has virtually no distinct flavor of its own and can be used in any dish while preserving the dish's own flavor profile. That's why it's our main go-to oil for all cooking and baking.

>> **Lard:** Lard has a bad reputation because it contains saturated fats. But lard has fewer saturated fats than butter. It also has about double the amount of healthy plant-based fats. Be sure to buy lard that is from free-range animals because it has the most nutritional benefits. While lard is typically made from pork fat, you can also try to find other animal fats like duck fat or tallow, all of which are minimally processed and tasty.

On the keto diet, most people stick to these three oils: olive oil, avocado oil, and coconut oil. In general, you want to avoid oils high in polyunsaturated fats, including corn oil, sunflower oil, soybean oil, safflower oil, and canola oil.

REMEMBER

Be cautious when choosing a solid fat. Some solid fats, like shortening, may contain artificial trans fats. Although shortening and lard may look similar at room temperature, they're very different in their fat contents. Try not to cook or bake with fats like shortening or stick margarine!

Slathering on the butter and mayo

This is the part of the keto diet that so many people enjoy. You can feel free to use all the full-fat mayo and creamy butter that you like! Do your best to purchase quality mayonnaise that is made with a good oil (avocado or olive oil), egg yolks, and vinegar. You can even try making your own mayonnaise from scratch, which is surprisingly easy to do.

Remember to look for butter produced from hormone-free, antibiotic-free cows. Always opt for butter rather than margarine. Margarine often has artificial trans fats, which have been associated with heart disease. Go for the real thing — the tasty, decadent butter.

REMEMBER

Ghee is a great alternative to butter. Ghee is simply clarified butter, which is butter that has been heated and had the milk solids removed. It may have a slightly nutty flavor from the heating process. Ghee can be used exactly like butter, and you can feel good about using it. Ghee has beneficial short- and medium-chain fatty acids and lots of healthy fats. Some studies have shown that ghee may even help improve your gut health.

Scoping out other great sources of healthy fats

We cover a lot of healthy fats in this chapter, but there are many more you can still scope out. Healthy, alternative fats are everywhere, and you will notice them more and more once you start looking from the keto point of view. Avocados, seeds, nuts, and soy-based proteins all have nutrients that help keep you feeling full and energized. Even tofu has healthy fats and proteins, and it is such a versatile food.

You have endless options when it comes to keto and fats. Cooking with extra fats and consuming delicious fats may be new to you after years of thinking fat was "bad," so now you have a whole, exciting food world to explore.

Grabbing low-carb veggies

Yes, the keto diet revolves around healthy fats, but you still need the other food groups to help you stay healthy. Vegetables are important to a well-balanced keto diet and help you get your recommended amount of fiber. Low-carb veggies are a great source of vitamins, minerals, and antioxidants. You want to load up on veggies just as much as you want to focus on fats.

Be sure to select veggies that are low in carbs. A good rule is to choose vegetables that grow above ground. Tubers and root vegetables tend to have the highest carbs. Some good vegetable options include:

>> Artichokes

>> Asparagus

>> Bell peppers

>> Broccoli

>> Cabbage

>> Cauliflower

>> Celery

- Cucumbers

- Garlic

- Leafy greens (kale, spinach, arugula, and so on)

- Onions

- Zucchini

REMEMBER

Try preparing your vegetables in different ways. Many veggies are delicious when simply chopped and served raw alongside a keto dip or sauce. Others are great to sauté or bake in a keto cooking oil. You'll never grow tired of eating vegetables if you prepare them in new and exciting ways. We provide a ton of recipes in this book to help you do just that!

Choosing low-glycemic fruits

We talk a little bit about the glycemic index in Chapter 3, so you may remember that low glycemic carbs are the ones that are less likely to increase your blood-sugar levels. While all fruits have natural sugars, you want to be sure to choose the fruits that have a low glycemic index to keep your blood sugar steady. Fruits do still have carbs, which contribute to your total daily carb count. While, yes, you can enjoy some fruits on a keto diet, you want to do so in moderation.

Here are a few of our favorite fruits that you can enjoy while still staying in ketosis:

- Berries (raspberries, blackberries, and strawberries, for example)

- Coconuts

- Lemons

- Limes

WHY FIBER DOESN'T COUNT

Whenever you look at the total carbs on the nutritional labels, it's a good rule of thumb to subtract the fiber because it doesn't truly count toward your daily carb intake. Although fiber is considered by the FDA to be a contributor toward total carbs, it doesn't get broken down into glucose like sugar and other carbohydrates. Fiber is listed separately from the total carb counts in Europe for exactly this reason. When you hear that the goal on a keto diet is 25 grams of carbs, it really means it's 25 grams of net carbs, which doesn't include fiber.

>> Tomatoes (yes, they're fruits!)

>> Watermelons (a few slices)

You can have a little bit of most other fruits. It's all about moderation. If you're making coleslaw salad, you can (and should) add half an apple. You can always look up how many grams of carbs a fruit has by typing in "fruit name + nutrition" on Google to determine how much you can have based on your daily carb allowance.

REMEMBER

Remember that buying high-quality fruits is very important. The fruit producers of the world tend to spray fruits with excess chemicals both to encourage growth and to preserve the fruits longer. Berries and tomatoes are fruits that you should always buy organic.

Choosing the best artificial sweeteners

The keto diet is known for focusing on the savory rather than the sweet, even though it's simply not true. Yes, you get to eat lots of fats and oils, but you will crave sweetness here and there like anyone else. After following a keto diet for a while, you will be surprised how your body adjusts and no longer looks for sweet foods; however, there are plenty of sweet options for you to enjoy once you know what to look for. The most important part of eating sweets on keto is making sure they were made with keto-safe sweeteners.

These are the sweeteners that are allowed on the keto diet:

>> **Stevia:** Stevia is a natural, sugar-like sweetener that has no calories or carbs. You can find stevia in powdered form or liquid. Studies have shown that stevia does not increase insulin levels, which makes it great for the keto diet. A little bit goes a long way when it comes to adding sweetness, so be sure to use a small amount. Stevia does have a slightly bitter aftertaste — another reason why you should only use a little bit at a time.

>> **Erythritol:** Erythritol is a sugar alcohol, but unlike other sugar alcohols, it does not increase insulin levels. Erythritol has virtually 0 calories but is about 70 percent as sweet as sugar. It acts, looks, and feels almost identical to sugar and is fantastic in drinks and baked goods. You can find plenty of keto beverages sold in stores that are made with erythritol. Another perk is that erythritol is good for your teeth.

>> **Xylitol:** Xylitol is another sugar alcohol that the body doesn't fully digest, meaning it doesn't spike insulin levels. Xylitol is just as sweet as sugar but with 40 percent fewer calories than sugar. Xylitol dissolves easily, making it great for mixing into your coffee or tea.

>> **Monk fruit:** Monk fruit sweetener, also known as "Lo Han Guo," comes from a small fruit in Southeast Asia. Monk fruit sweetener has no calories, no carbs, and is about 200 to 500 times sweeter than sugar. The intense sweetness in monk fruit sweetener comes from mogrosides. It's often combined with erythritol to make a sweetener that's as sweet as sugar (erythritol alone is 70 percent as sweet as sugar).

>> **Allulose:** Allulose is a rare sugar that occurs naturally in some foods like wheat, figs, and raisins. Like erythritol, it's about 70 percent as sweet as sugar. It's also virtually calorie free. Both allulose and erythritol are now considered the best sugar replacements commercially, so you'll see plenty of keto products on store shelves using either of the two or both together.

TIP

Each sweetener has its own benefits and unique sweetness, so some people like to mix them together. Mixing sweeteners can also help achieve baked goods that are the right consistency and taste. Try experimenting a little with mixing sweeteners when you bake and cook. One popular combination is stevia and erythritol.

Using Common Replacements for Keto

You probably have a few recipes that you love to make. It can be hard to give up those favorites if these recipes are not keto-approved. However, there are ways you can tweak your recipes to fit the keto diet just by making a few simple changes.

There are lots of substitutes you can use for carb-heavy ingredients like flour or sugar. When you have a grasp on the substitutes and common replacements you can use, you'll be able to take almost any recipe and adjust it to fit your diet. Your favorite recipes will be saved!

Keto-friendly replacements for flour

One of the first ingredients you need to ditch when starting a keto diet is flour. Classic white flour is almost all carbs and has little nutritional value. Substituting flour for alternatives not only makes your recipes keto-friendly, but also make them healthier overall. Following are a few of our favorite keto-friendly flour alternatives and how to use them.

Almond flour and nut flours

Almond flour is one of the best grain-free alternatives to wheat flour. It is low in carbs and has lots of healthy fats and protein. Almond flour is made by finely grinding whole, blanched almonds. You can easily make your own almond flour, but you can also find it in most grocery stores.

Since almond flour is much higher in fat than regular flour, it bakes a little differently than wheat flour, making foods that are much denser. Use a little less oil or butter in your recipes when replacing wheat flour with nut flour. You may also want to add an extra egg to your baked goods to help provide more structure. Adding extra rising agents, like more baking powder, also helps.

Coconut flour

Coconut flour is made from dehydrated coconut meat. Most of the fat is removed from the coconut before the flour is made, which makes the coconut flour soft and light, just like wheat flours. However, baking with coconut flour is still very different from baking with wheat flour. Coconut flour soaks up liquids, making baked goods very dense and chewy.

For every 1 cup of wheat flour in a recipe, use ⅓ cup of coconut flour instead. You also want to add about two to three extra eggs to help baked goods hold together. These changes can be quite drastic to a recipe, so you may want to search for recipes that use coconut flour initially rather than use it as a substitute.

Ground flax meal

Ground flaxseeds can be used as a flour in baking and cooking. However, due to its earthy taste, flax meal is best used as a secondary flour in baking. A mix of ground flaxseeds and almond flour, for example, works well. Try replacing 1 cup of wheat flour with ½ cup almond flour and ¼ cup of ground flaxseeds.

Flaxseeds are high in vitamins and omega-3 fatty acids. They do have carbs, but they are mostly from fiber.

Sunflower seed meal

Ground sunflower seeds make a fluffy, light flour. Seed flours are very high in vitamins and minerals like vitamin E. They are also low in carbs. They are a good flour substitute for anyone with a nut allergy.

You can replace almond flour in a recipe with the same quantity of sunflower meal, making any recipe nut free. Almond flour and sunflower meal have many of the same properties and bake in the same way.

REMEMBER

Keto baking can be tricky, especially when you start using alternative flours. These wheat-flour replacements can work very well when used correctly. Trying to convert one of your favorite recipes into a keto-safe version can be a trial-and-error process. Don't give up! Play around with keto flours and you'll quickly get the hang of how they work.

Keto-friendly replacements for cow's milk

Milk contains lactose, a natural sugar. We talk earlier about how full-fat milk has less lactose, making it a better substitute for low-fat milks. There are also some great nondairy options as well. Milk alternatives can add a lot of extra vitamins and minerals to your recipes too.

Here are a few of our favorite keto milks:

>> **Unsweetened coconut milk:** Coconut milk is naturally sweet, which many people love. Some types are thicker than others depending on the fat content. Coconut milk is high in healthy fats. It adds a nice taste to recipes and is also good to drink on its own.

>> **Almond milk:** Almond milk is a great plant-based milk. It is creamy and rich with a slight nutty taste. To make almond milk, whole almonds are soaked in water, blended, and then strained through a cheesecloth. You can buy unsweetened almond milk or make your own.

>> **Soy milk:** Soy milk is made from soaking soybeans in water and then grinding and straining them to make a smooth liquid. Soy milk has a generally neutral taste, so it is good with sweet or savory foods. Some people prefer other milk alternatives over soy milk since soy is often genetically modified. However, it's still a good nondairy substitute.

When choosing your milk alternative, be sure to always pick unsweetened milks. Many almond milks and coconut milks have flavors and sweeteners that you want to avoid. You can also try making your own nut milks at home. They are quite easy and satisfying to make.

Changing Your Beverage Options

Choosing the right beverages can have a huge impact on your keto diet and your overall health. Many Americans drink a large percentage of their carbs by consuming lots of sugar-sweetened beverages. You may be surprised how many carbs you can cut from your diet just by adjusting your beverage choices.

Drinking water is so important

Water is always the best drink, no matter what diet you are following. This is especially important for keto dieters because your body utilizes water to burn fat. As you use the water in your body to convert fats to energy, through a process called *lipolysis*, you need to replace that water to keep your body working efficiently and feeling good.

We know that it can be hard to drink enough water. Water has a neutral taste, so it's not something you likely crave. However, water is essential! Here are a few tips and tricks to help you drink more water and enjoy every sip.

Flavor your water with fruits and herbs

Flavorless, plain water isn't always appealing. Adding a little flavor to the water can make it taste better and be a little more interesting. A simple slice of lemon is always a good idea. You can also add a small handful of berries or some sprigs of mint or even rosemary to your glass. Always be sure to use fresh, clean fruits and herbs. Be sure they are also keto! You don't want hidden carbs sneaking into your water glass.

Add a no- or low-calorie water enhancer

You can find water-enhancing drops that add flavor and sweetness to your water without carbs or calories. Everly water enhancer is a natural, stevia-sweetened drink mix made with vegetable juices. Star Liquid water enhancer is another stevia-sweetened, calorie-free flavor addition that really livens up your water. Be sure to look at the ingredient list of every water enhancer to make sure it is completely keto safe.

Keep your water cold

Cold water is much more refreshing and satisfying than room temperature water for a lot of people. You are more likely to enjoy chilled water and, therefore, drink more of it.

REMEMBER

Most people need between 11 and 16 cups of beverages per day. Most of this should be consumed in water. This number can be daunting, but once you start drinking the right amount of water, you will notice how good you feel. Being well-hydrated can help reduce headaches, improve the appearance of your skin, and help your muscles and joints work better. And once you're in the swing of things and your body is used to getting enough water, you'll notice your body asking for water almost every hour.

Avoiding zero-calorie soft drinks

Many sodas and soft drinks may claim they have zero calories, but research has shown that they are still very likely to cause weight gain and long-term health issues. The artificial sweeteners in most soft drinks can still cause insulin production, causing inflammation and buildup in your bloodstream. Diet sodas tend to use the worst kind of artificial sweeteners and other unhealthy ingredients, which have been linked to health outcomes such as osteoporosis and headaches.

TIP

There are quite a few keto-friendly energy drinks that are much better than diet sodas. If you are tired of water or looking for a little caffeinated pick-me-up, try one of these drinks instead:

>> **Bai:** These drinks are sweetened with erythritol and usually contain 1 or 2 grams of net carbs per bottle. Don't drink more than one a day, though, because the erythritol servings are quite high, which can cause some bloating or gassiness.

>> **Powerade Zero:** This drink has beneficial electrolytes and none of the carbs found in regular Powerade. It is made with sucralose, which doesn't raise your glucose levels. It is also very sweet despite having no real sugar. It can keep you hydrated and satisfy a sweet-tooth craving.

>> **Zero Calorie Vitamin Water:** This energy drink is made with stevia and erythritol, two keto-approved sweeteners. It also provides about 25 percent of your daily zinc requirements. It's a good soda alternative.

>> **Wave Soda Sparkling Juice:** This low-calorie, caffeine-filled drink boosts your energy and keeps you refreshed. It is a good option if you want a sweet drink without the carbs. These drinks still have some sugar due to the juice content, so you shouldn't have these too often.

>> **Hint Water:** Hint is a bottled, fruit-infused water that has no carbs and no sugar. It is a great option if you want fruit water on the go. There are lots of flavor options you can try so you'll never get bored of this tasty drink.

Grabbing a bottle of cold water is always the best idea. However, here and there, bottled drinks can be a nice change in your routine. Always make sure they use keto-approved sweeteners and are truly low in net carbs after subtracting the sugar alcohols and/or fiber from the total carb number.

Chapter **5**

Getting to Know Your Macros

The term "macros" is short for macronutrients. These are the main chemical elements that your body needs to thrive. The macros that our diets revolve around are fats, carbs, and protein.

The keto diet is based heavily around fats. It requires a moderate amount of protein and very few carbs. Becoming familiar with these macros is important as it helps you succeed on a keto diet. In this chapter, we show you how to really assess macronutrients by reading the nutrition label to see the true value in every food. By the end of the chapter, you'll be a macro pro!

Calculating Macro Targets

The keto diet is not just about calories but also about the total number of macronutrients you consume. You need to know how much of each macro you are consuming throughout the day to stay in ketosis. People are not very good at guessing macros, calories, or even a true portion size of a meal. This is especially true since portion sizes have dramatically increased in the last few decades.

If you underestimate the number of calories and carbs you are eating, you may have a hard time losing weight and/or gaining any real benefits from the keto diet. You need to know the real numbers to be successful. You also need to be very in tune with what you are eating throughout the day. You may remember to calculate the macros of your main meals but forget to add in those little snacks you eat between meals. These need to be accounted for as well as any beverages you drink that may have carbs.

We give you a few tools to help you determine your real macro numbers rather than relying on inaccurate "guesstimates." There are also a lot of fantastic macro calculators that we recommend using. A simple app can do wonders for keeping track of your daily fats, proteins, and carbs.

Determining total calories

Total calories are the number of calories your body needs every day to produce enough energy to carry out its essential functions. This number is also called the *resting metabolic rate* (RMR). You need a certain number of calories just to breathe, rest, and create new cells. Your personal RMR is unique to you because the number of calories your body needs varies greatly based on your weight, body mass, age, activity level, and even your gender. People who are more active need more calories. People who are taller also have higher caloric needs. Exposure to temperature fluctuations also jump-starts your RMR because your body needs to regulate itself to the rise and fall of weather conditions. So many things affect how many calories your body needs.

What you eat affects your metabolism. Starvation diets decrease your metabolism because your body starts trying to conserve energy, knowing it isn't getting more calories any time soon. Your metabolism can drop by as much as 30 percent when you cut calories too quickly. This can, in turn, make it harder to lose weight. Eating less food rapidly is not the answer to weight loss!

You can determine your personal RMR in two ways: indirect calorimetry and RMR calculators.

Indirect calorimetry

Indirect calorimetry is a very accurate way to determine your RMR, but it is also time consuming and expensive. *Indirect calorimetry* measures the amount of heat your body produces by calculating how much carbon dioxide and nitrogen you exhale. These two gasses are the end products of metabolism, so they can indicate how your metabolism is working in a given time period.

A personal trainer, doctor, or nutritionist can help you do an indirect calorimetry test. You breathe into a device that measures your breath and gives you an RMR reading.

RMR Calculators

RMR calculators use complex formulas that use several criteria to come up with the number of calories you should eat per day. Many of the calculators are great at determining your basal caloric needs, but based on external varying factors, the calories can be off by almost 300 per day. That's enough to cause a weight change of about a pound a week! These calculators are good to give you a general idea of the calorie count your body needs, but you should always keep in mind that they are not the most accurate.

If you are serious about your keto diet and want to ensure you're successful, you may want to consider having an indirect calorimetry test done. It can give you a great grasp on the calories you need to help you maintain or lose weight and stay healthy throughout your keto journey.

REMEMBER

Dieticians and nutritionists like to use the Mifflin-St. Jeor equation to calculate RMR. It is a time-tested equation that can often get your RMR within a 50-calorie range. That's pretty accurate!

Keep in mind that the more physical activity you do, the more calories your body needs. You need to modify your daily caloric intake based on activity.

You also need to apply your weight loss goals to your daily caloric intake number. If you are trying to gain weight, your calorie intake should go up. If the goal is to lose weight, your calorie intake should go down. Do not shift these numbers drastically, though, as that can have a negative impact. A good rule of thumb is to cut about 250 calories per day to lose half a pound per week and not feel like you're starving yourself.

The basic math for weight loss starts with your RMR number, adds the amount of physical activity you do, and matches this with what you eat. Lots of online calculators use the Mifflin-St. Jeor equation to give you a good number of calories you should be eating each day. We strongly recommend using this tool to get started.

REMEMBER

It's is a good idea to reassess your RMR after about every 5 pounds you lose. Don't worry, though! Just because you need to eat less doesn't mean you will start to be hungry more often. Your body needs less, and your appetite will reflect this as well.

CALORIC DEFICITS AND KETO: HOW THEY WORK TOGETHER

A caloric deficit means eating fewer calories than your body burns. This is a cornerstone of weight loss and what people do when they are trying to shed pounds. Cutting too many calories can have the opposite effect, causing your metabolism to drop as your body tries to ration energy. However, having a slight caloric deficit, even on a keto diet, will help you lose weight.

On a keto diet, the body is burning more fats as fuel than you consume and, in turn, using fat stores for energy. There is no starvation or drastic drop in calories. A keto diet limits calories in targeted ways, helping you lose weight while still getting enough energy through food and stored fat, while avoiding the breakdown of muscles for extra energy.

Realizing the importance of the high fat, moderate protein, and low carb balance

You know that high fat, moderate protein, and low carb is the goal of keto, but getting the proper balance of these macronutrients is just as important. You need to stick to the percentages and numbers of your customized keto diet to achieve success.

When in ketosis, your body burns fats as fuel. This is why your fat intake is so high; this is where your body is getting the majority of its energy. Protein is still very important. Every cell in the human body contains protein, and you need protein to repair your cells as well as make new ones. However, you want to keep your carbs very low and never consume more than your allotted daily intake. The moment you consume more carbs, your body will snatch them up and use them as energy, abandoning all those healthy fats you have been eating and kicking you out of ketosis.

Carbs (glucose) are much easier to process as a source of energy, and they're dangerous if they're sitting around in your bloodstream for too long. That's why your body must create insulin to help your cells absorb the glucose in your blood and reduce it to a normal, manageable level. And once it prioritizes the glucose for energy to avoid what is basically glucose toxicity, it will need less from the fats you've eaten. If your body gets everything it needs calorie-wise from carbs, it'll choose to store away the fats instead. That's why macronutrient balance is key!

REMEMBER

Know your macronutrient numbers and keep track of them using an app like Total Keto Diet. Keep your diet balanced to gain all the benefits from keto. Always ask your doctor or healthcare provider if you are concerned about your diet. Your personal plan needs to fit your unique life, and your situation may always be changing. Keto is very flexible, but you need to come up with *your* keto plan and then stick to it!

WARNING

Some women stick to a keto diet throughout pregnancy and breastfeeding. However, it's not a good idea to start your keto journey while pregnant or breast-feeding. Drastic dietary changes of any kind are not advised during pregnancy unless directed by a doctor. Pregnancy causes a wide array of changes to your body, and adding extreme dietary changes on top of that may not be the best idea and may lead to unintended consequences for the mother and baby.

The effects of excess ketones on a fetus have yet to really be explored. While some hypothesize the ketones may help child development, other studies suggest that ketones may have a negative impact on the fetus. Pregnancy and breastfeeding are rare times when ketoacidosis may also occur even if a person does not have diabetes. A mother's body is so metabolically active during this time that ketoaci-dosis may be triggered.

The bottom line is new mothers who are already following a keto diet may be able to safely continue a keto lifestyle throughout pregnancy. It is not recommended to begin a keto diet while pregnant or while breastfeeding. Or course, you should always consult your doctor and discuss any dietary needs or concerns, especially when pregnant.

Net carbs versus total carbs

There are three different types of carbs:

>> Complex carbohydrates like starches

>> Simple carbohydrates like sugar

>> Indigestible carbohydrates like fiber and sugar alcohols

A nutrition label adds up all those carbs and lists the number of total carbs in a food.

Your body absorbs and uses the complex and simple carbs, increasing your carb intake greatly. These two types of carbs collectively need to be kept under a 25- to 30-gram-per-day limit or they'll kick you out of ketosis. The indigestible carbs, on the other hand, go right through your system, helping improve gut health and keeping your body regular. These indigestible carbs are highly encouraged even on a keto diet. Because the body can't digest most types of fiber, it doesn't use fiber as glucose or increase your insulin levels, making it great for the keto lifestyle.

Total carbohydrates are the sum of all the carbs in a food. Net carbs are what you get when you subtract all the nondigestible carbs coming from fiber and sugar alcohols. When you remove the nondigestible carbs that the body doesn't actually absorb, you are left with the net carb amount, which is the actual number of carbs that remain in your body and are turned into glucose.

When you look at a nutrition label, find the total carb number and then subtract the fiber and sugar alcohols like erythritol and allulose. You'll find that many keto products sold in stores use both fiber and sugar alcohols.

Net Carbs = Total Carbs – Fiber – Sugar Alcohols

This net carb number is the one you really want to focus on when on a keto diet.

TYPES OF FIBER AND HOW YOU BENEFIT FROM THEM

Fiber is an important part of your diet. Eating fiber has many benefits, including maintaining your digestive health, lowering triglyceride and cholesterol levels, and keeping you full longer, which helps with weight loss.

Soluble fiber dissolves in water to form a gel-like substance and helps to slow down digestion in your stomach. Soluble fiber can be found in foods like bananas, Brussels sprouts, avocados, beans, peas, and apples.

Insoluble fiber doesn't dissolve in water but remains whole as it passes through your stomach, helping keep your bowels healthy and regular. It's found in foods like nuts, seeds, and skins of fruits and vegetables.

Most Americans get only half their daily recommended fiber, and that's easily fixable on the keto diet. Many foods that are non-keto like bread or wraps are made keto by switching out high-carb ingredients like flour with fiber-based flours. Eating even one keto wrap usually covers your daily fiber needs.

Personalizing Keto Goals

You are probably thinking about how great it will be to dive right into a keto diet. But before you jump in headfirst, you should ask yourself one important question: "What do I want to gain from following a keto diet?"

Keto is more than just a trendy diet; it is a lifestyle. It is training your body to eat and produce energy in a whole new way. We have already gone over the many benefits of the keto diet, and you are probably drawn to more than one of them. But what outcome of the keto diet are you most excited about?

>> Do you want to lose weight?

>> Are you discouraged by other diets and think keto will fit your life better?

>> Are you excited about delicious keto foods?

>> Do you want to build muscle or get more toned?

>> Are you trying to treat high cholesterol or prevent heart disease?

>> Are you looking to prevent long-term illnesses like obesity or diabetes?

There are so many reasons why keto may be perfect for you; setting real goals will help you customize the keto diet to fit your needs.

TIP

Many people find it helpful to write down their goals. You can keep these goals in a safe place, and anytime you are struggling on the keto diet, take out your goals and recommit. It will help you greatly, especially in the first few weeks when your body is transitioning into ketosis.

Combining keto, your current lifestyle, and the lifestyle you want

Are you a super athlete? Or maybe you are more of a couch person. No matter your current lifestyle, you can incorporate keto into your routine and make it work for you.

Assessing your current activity levels is important when starting the keto diet. You need to look at how active you are and decide how active you would like to be. Keto diets do work well in conjunction with exercise. However, like we said before, you don't have to be a star athlete to benefit from keto.

When you start planning for your keto diet, decide what kind of lifestyle you want. Do you want to start running five days a week, or does just a walk around the block sound nice? If you plan to hit the gym every day, this can work too. Commit to your activity level just as you are committing to the keto diet.

Next, calculate your daily caloric intake with your planned activity levels using an online calculator or keto app. This gives you true numbers that can help drive the success of your diet. Remember to always be realistic about the lifestyle you want. You know yourself best, and you know how much activity you will really do. Be honest and truthful when you set your goals. The keto diet can work for anyone, so there is no reason to pretend you will start marathon training when you will just be sitting down for a movie marathon on your couch. Real numbers, regardless of what they are, give you real success.

REMEMBER

Remember to always reassess your caloric intake and macronutrient numbers every so often. Your weight, activity levels, and age will all change as you go along your keto journey. Even little changes, like dropping a pound or two, affect your diet.

Make a plan to calculate your macros once a month. Set a reminder in your phone so you won't forget. Use an app or an easy online calculator to make it simple and straightforward. Be sure to keep track of the results so you know what your current macronutrient goals are.

Targeting specific health conditions

The keto diet has been shown to help many different health conditions, from diabetes to epilepsy. Knowing how beneficial keto can be to your health is a big motivator when it comes to sticking to the keto diet.

One of the biggest reasons why people choose keto other than for weight loss is to help control blood-sugar levels. Type 2 diabetes occurs because the body has been exposed to high levels of glucose and insulin for so long that the insulin no longer does its job. Insulin resistance and insulin insensitivity are the result, and blood sugar rises even if insulin levels are high. Type 2 diabetes is often called adult-onset diabetes as people tend to suffer from this disease later in life. However, now many younger people are getting type 2 diabetes because of eating carb-loaded snacks and foods.

The classic low-fat-and-high-carb diet does not help with blood sugar levels, but many nutritionists and doctors have praised the effects of the keto diet when it comes to controlling type 2 diabetes.

If you want to get the full benefits of the keto diet regarding blood-sugar levels, you must be sure to fully commit to the diet. A modified keto diet doesn't work well in this scenario, but the standard keto diet does. Stick with your macro numbers and you will see quite the improvement in the way you feel.

We talk previously about all the conditions that a keto diet can help. Here is a refresher on health issues that keto may help prevent, cure, or reduce:

» Bad cholesterol and triglyceride levels

» Acne and skin conditions

» Insomnia

» Seizures and epilepsy

» Neurodegenerative diseases like Alzheimer's disease

» Migraines and headaches

» Fibromyalgia

» Polycystic ovary syndrome (PCOS)

» Chronic inflammation

The keto diet has also been shown to help people with cardiovascular disease and chronic pain. If you often feel tired, foggy, or just generally under the weather, the keto diet can help by boosting your energy levels in a healthy way.

When people think of "diets," weight loss immediately comes to mind. While yes, the keto diet can help with weight loss, it can do so much more. There are so many reasons why you may benefit from the keto diet that it just makes sense to give it a try. You don't have much to lose!

REMEMBER

You should always consult your doctor before jumping into a new diet, especially one that will have a drastic change on your body as the keto diet surely will. This is especially true if you are already taking medication to lower your blood sugar. The keto diet is so low in carbs that this, combined with blood-sugar-dropping medications, may make your sugar levels dangerously low.

Vindicating dietary fat

While eating carbs may be the way you fuel your body now, carbohydrates are not actually an essential macronutrient. You can survive without carbs. Fat, on the other hand is essential, and you need it to live. Fat is imperative for a well-functioning body. It helps your brain signals fire smoothly; it is part of cell development; and it is fundamental in hormone development, which the body needs to thrive. If we didn't have fats in our diet, our system would struggle to complete basic functions, which could lead to chronic illness, inflammation, obesity, and more. Fat is important! It is not the villain that the modern food industry has made it out to be.

REMEMBER Your body needs fat to function. Contrary to popular myth, fat does not make you fat. Excess calories are what lead to weight gain and health issues. Fats are our friends, but like anything else, overdoing it on the calories is when you run into issues, whether it be on a high-carb or a high-fat diet.

Upping your consumption of healthy fats

Once you have figured out how many total calories you need, it's time to look at how much of each macronutrient you need. Fat, of course is a big one on the keto diet. You need to decide which type of keto diet you will be following, but if you're like most of us, you will probably start with the standard keto diet where 70 to 75 percent of calories should come from fats, 20 to 25 percent from protein, and 5 percent from carbs.

Here is a look at the fat consumption numbers (at 75 percent) for a person on a 2,000-calorie diet:

2,000 x 0.75 = 1,500 calories from fat per day

Unfortunately, most nutrition labels only tell you the amount of nutrients listed in grams. There are 9 calories in every gram of fat. So, 1,500 calories from fat means you need to consume

1,500/9 = 167 grams of fat per day.

REMEMBER Remember that your fat and protein intake will vary slightly based on the keto diet you are following. Those on a medical keto diet, one that controls epilepsy, may need up to 80 percent fat per day. Someone following a protein keto diet may only require 65 percent fat. The keto diet is completely customized to fit your needs, so be aware that your numbers and formulas may be slightly different.

Calculating your protein target

Now that you know how to calculate required fats from calories, you can easily figure out how much protein your body needs. If you are following a keto diet that dictates 20 percent calories should come from protein on a 2,000-calorie diet, you will need

2,000 x 0.2 = 400 calories from protein per day

Protein is one of the building blocks of life. It is necessary for healthy brain function, cell production, skin and bone health, and building muscle mass. You will consume plenty of protein on a keto diet, but you want to be sure not to overdo it.

Eating protein doesn't affect your ketone levels. However, too much protein can cause excess gluconeogenesis (GNG). GNG is a metabolic pathway that allows your liver to make glucose from non-carb sources, which is what happens on keto to maintain stable glucose levels. Many people worry that excess protein will turn into glucose via GNG. The truth is that this won't affect ketosis unless you're eating double to triple your recommended protein amount.

The main reason why you don't want to consume too much protein is so that your main source of calories is still fats. Fats are the key to energy on the keto diet, and you want to be sure you are getting enough of them. If you start eating too much protein, your fat intake will naturally go down and you will feel the effects. High fats, moderate protein, and low carbs is the best balance for ketosis.

There are 4 calories in every gram of protein, which means you need

400/4 = 100 grams of protein per day

If you are trying to bulk up and increase muscle, you will need about 1 gram of protein per pound of lean body weight. Our calculations here are based on maintaining muscle rather than increasing it.

REMEMBER

Try to focus on losing excess fat before building muscle. Building muscle and really bulking up requires extra calories. You don't want to be increasing your calorie count before you achieve your weight goals. It can be quite complicated to try to balance losing weight and having enough calories to build muscle. Focus on one at a time and you will be more successful.

Slashing your carb intake

Your total carb intake goes way, way down on the keto diet. This is the macro that requires the least number of calories. A standard keto diet requires about 5 percent of your daily caloric intake to be from carbs. If you are on a 2,000-calorie diet, this means

2,000 x .05 = 100 calories of carbohydrates per day.

Take those 100 calories and determine the total grams of carbs by dividing by 4. There are 4 calories in every gram of carb.

100/4 = 25 grams of carbs per day

Twenty-five grams of carbs per day is a good place to start when you begin your keto journey. Some people may be able to stay in ketosis while consuming more carbs (people who work out a lot can consume around 50 grams of carbs per day on average) while others may need to cut the carb count even further. This all depends on what your body can handle. A targeted keto diet may also require a few extra carbs to fuel you through some hard physical exercise. All in all, this formula is a great jumping-off point.

REMEMBER

Knowing your daily caloric intake and the calories needed from each macronutrient is essential to keto. You need to know these numbers to be successful. So, dust off that old calculator to keep track of your numbers or find yourself a new app to guide you. Any tools that can help you are wonderful!

WARNING

Alcohol is also technically a macronutrient and contains 7 calories per gram, but because it's not essential for survival, it's not mentioned with the other macros. However, it is important to keep those calories in mind when consuming alcohol. Even pure, hard liquor is around 100 calories per shot, meaning calories from alcohol add up quick. Keep that in mind when you're counting calories or trying to lose weight.

Chapter **6**

Eating Out on Keto

O ne of the most exciting parts of the keto diet is discovering how to cook healthy, nutritious meals for yourself. Keto can really push you in the kitchen, requiring you to take charge of your meals to hit your macronutrients goals. It is also quite satisfying to know that you prepared a meal all on your own and that it is something you can thoroughly enjoy. Sitting down to dinner has never felt so good!

But every now and then, you may need a day off. We all deserve a little break from cooking, and the chance to have someone else prepare a meal for us is too good to pass up.

The idea of dining out should be exciting rather than stressful. You should never feel anxiety about sticking to your keto goals while at a restaurant. You just need to know how to order, how to avoid carbs, and how to get the best meal possible without ruining your hard keto work.

In this chapter, we help you navigate the restaurant menu so that you can enjoy your night out. The keto diet is full of fantastic foods, and there are sure to be restaurants near you that can cater to your keto lifestyle.

Choosing Keto-Friendly Restaurants

Almost every restaurant has something keto friendly on the menu, even if it requires a slight adjustment. From thick cuts of meat to delicious morning omelets at a diner, you are bound to find something you can enjoy eating guilt-free. You may need to adjust dishes slightly, skipping a sauce or swapping pasta for a salad, but when you know what to look for in the menu description, you'll know what to avoid.

TIP

Look at the restaurant's menu online ahead of time. You can likely tell with just a quick glance if there are keto-friendly foods for you. You can also try calling the restaurant beforehand and asking about low-carb dishes. Restaurants are part of the hospitality industry, so they want customers to be happy. They should be more than willing to answer any dietary questions you may have.

Some types of cuisines are naturally better for those on a keto diet. While a popular pasta restaurant may be one you want to skip, your local steakhouse may have lots of delicious menu items for you to try.

Steakhouses and BBQ restaurants

Steakhouses and BBQ joints are a keto dieter's paradise. These establishments have thick, juicy pieces of fatty meats prepared in tons of different ways. Even if you must ditch the sauce, a steakhouse likely knows how to properly cook a great cut of meat. You may only need a sprinkle of sea salt to accompany a good cut of steak that is prepared well.

Steakhouses and barbecue restaurants often have good veggie side dishes. They do tend to have lots of potato-based sides as well, which you need to skip. Coleslaw, on the other hand, is a barbecue restaurant special that is likely to be keto approved. Just ask whether any sugar is added to the mix, which may be more often than you think. Be sure to ask about all sauces as lots of them have sugar added to the recipe, especially barbecue sauce.

Burgers are another popular menu item at American-style restaurants. A burger is very keto-friendly if you hold the bun and the ketchup. Many restaurants will replace the bun with a big piece of lettuce as a wrap. Feel free to load up on the mayonnaise and mustard; they're both keto-approved!

Buffets

Buffets revolve around catering to everyone's personal tastes. They offer a little of everything so that anyone who visits a buffet can find something they like. Many common keto items are on a standard buffet that you should be able to freely enjoy.

Breakfast buffets should have lots of egg-based options for you to choose from. Look for an omelet station where you can customize your own breakfast omelet or go right for the scrambled eggs.

Grilled steak, chicken, and fish are usually lightly seasoned and free of carbs. A salad bar at a buffet provides you with plenty of customizable options. Look for higher-fat salad add-ins such as shredded cheese, nuts, and avocado.

REMEMBER

Buffets can be dangerous when it comes to portion sizes. When you can scoop freely from large platters of food, it's very easy to take too much. One good rule of thumb is to make sure nothing on your plate touches. Keep portions small enough so they all have space on the plate. You can always go up to the buffet to get more if needed, but starting off small is a good idea. This also prevents you from eating too quickly and feeling stuffed and miserable after binging on buffet food.

Seafood

Seafood restaurants are very good options for those on a keto diet. Not only do you get a good dose of omega-3 fatty acids when you eat fish, but you're likely to find a good number of keto choices, giving you plenty of options to satisfy any food cravings.

Remember to skip any breaded fish dishes. Look for grilled, steamed, or broiled options instead. Be sure to ask for more cream sauce or some extra garlic butter to really make your keto dream dinner come true.

REMEMBER

Many seafood restaurants serve seafood with pasta or rice. These, of course, are no good for any keto dieter. If your seafood dish comes with a heavy, carb-loaded starch, ask for extra veggies instead. Most restaurants are more than willing to substitute pasta for a keto-friendly side.

Mediterranean

Mediterranean cuisine stems from various countries around the Mediterranean Sea such as Spain, Italy, Greece, Turkey, and Israel. The foods tend to be slathered in olive oil (yum!) and cooked in healthy, fresh ways using minimal ingredients.

Fresh bread is often a staple of the Mediterranean diet but is usually served as a side dish, so you can easily avoid it.

Most Mediterranean restaurants have lots of fresh fish, lamb, or chicken options. Fresh lemon juice, vinegar, and herbs are typically used as seasonings, and all are appropriate for the keto diet. You rarely find super-sweet, processed, or carb-loaded sauces in a Mediterranean restaurant, which is perfect for keto dieters.

Chinese

Chinese food can be tricky on a keto diet, but it can be doable. You just need to be aware of the sauces, which are too often sweetened with sugar and thickened with starch (another carb). Ask for your Chinese food to be prepared or served without sauce (or sauce on the side) to avoid any hidden carbs. Be sure to also skip any noodle dishes or rice.

Chinese food is often pan-fried and cooked quickly, which helps retain vitamins and minerals. You may also find roasted duck, chicken wings, steamed shrimp, pork ribs, and fresh Bok choy or broccoli on the menu — all fantastic keto options.

REMEMBER

Skip any hoisin, duck, oyster, sweet and sour, or plum sauce. All these sauces are made with an enormous amount of sugar and starch, which may sabotage your keto goals.

Japanese

Fresh seafood and fermented foods are both hallmarks of Japanese cuisine and are keto friendly. Seaweed salad and some seared fresh fish sounds like a dream! Just be aware that Japanese food is heavily focused on rice. Rice may come with almost every dish at your local Japanese restaurant, so be prepared to let your server know to hold the rice to avoid temptation.

Edamame is another Japanese classic that is one of those veggies that isn't good for keto diets. Edamame is high in carbs with ½ cup of the little beans containing around 9 grams of carbs. Skip the rice and the edamame, and you should be just fine at a Japanese restaurant.

REMEMBER

Choose sashimi, which is made without rice, over sushi. Or try asking if the restaurant can make sushi rolls without the rice. Since rolls are usually made to order, this can be a good option.

Avoiding Unnecessary Carbs and Maximizing Healthy Fats

The hardest part about eating at a restaurant is avoiding the hidden carbs. When you're not in charge of cooking the foods, you just don't know what ingredients are being used. Condiments, sauces, and side dishes are often the biggest culprits of hidden carbs. Here are a few ingredients that you always want to avoid no matter what type of restaurant or cuisine you are enjoying.

>> **Bread and breading:** The keto diet doesn't allow bread (unless it's marketed as a keto-friendly bread, oftentimes using almond flour). Skip the breadbasket on the table and avoid any menu items that are breaded and fried. Ask your server how your dish is prepared so you won't be surprised when your chicken comes out with a crispy bread coating.

REMEMBER

No matter the type of cuisine, you should always skip foods that are breaded because you know those breadcrumbs have a lot of carbs. If you order a Caesar salad, ask the kitchen to hold the croutons. Skip the rolls that are served at the beginning of the meal and ask for any burgers to be served without the buns.

>> **Potatoes:** From mashed potatoes to French fries, this is a starch you should skip. If your meal comes with fries, ask for a keto-approved, veggie side dish instead.

>> **Pasta, noodles, and rice:** Carb, carb, carb. Ask for your food to be served on a bed of fresh greens rather than a bed of carbs.

>> **Thick sauces:** Lots of thicker sauces are made thick by adding a starch such as cornstarch or flour. If you are ordering a meal that comes with a sauce, be sure to ask about the ingredients in the sauce. Barbecue sauce and teriyaki sauce are both red flags for a secretly high-carb meal, so try to avoid them.

>> **Condiments:** Ketchup is a popular condiment that you need to ditch when you start a keto diet. It has lots of sugar — both added into the recipe and naturally occurring in the tomatoes. Look for lower-carb condiments like mayonnaise, tabasco, coconut aminos, or mustard.

REMEMBER

Look for unsweetened condiments like mayonnaise, mustard, soy sauce, guacamole, pico de gallo, or white wine vinegar. If something is called "honey" mustard or "sweet" soy sauce, skip it.

>> **Balsamic vinegar:** Balsamic vinegar has a surprisingly high number of carbs. Other vinegars, like red wine vinegar, are good substitutes for balsamic. Skip any balsamic glaze–drenched salads as well.

- » **Sriracha:** Did you know that sriracha sauce is made of about 20 percent added sugar? That's why it has that sweet and spicy taste that so many people love. Look for a sugar-free Sriracha brand, which should be more keto friendly than the standard sauce.

- » **Desserts:** When dining out, you should probably skip dessert completely. Some restaurants may offer low-carb, sugar-free, or keto-friendly desserts, but this is rare. A cheese plate or bowl of fresh berries may be a good option in place of a classic dessert.

Now that you are well versed in how to avoid carbs when dining out, consider how to maximize healthy fats. Fats and proteins should be the main part of your restaurant meal, just like when you are at home. Here are a few delicious fats you should look for on the restaurant menu:

- » **Butter:** Ask your server for extra butter or oil. You can use it on your meats and veggies to add some extra fat to your restaurant meal. Some restaurants have fantastic infused oils or specialty butters that are worth trying.

- » **Cheese:** Anything made with hard cheese can be perfect for the keto diet. Maybe your local restaurant has a cheese platter you'd like to try. Cheeses and their accompaniments can be a complete meal!

- » **Creamy sauces:** A cream sauce is perfect for anyone on a keto diet. The rich butter and cream are hearty, fatty, and delicious. Ask for extra cream sauces so you can pour them over your meats and veggies to enhance your dining experience. You may want to ask if the restaurant thickens their cream sauce with flour or another starch. Most don't because cream sauces are thick enough on their own, but it's always good practice to ask!

- » **Eggs:** Eggs are a keto dieter's best friend. Luckily, there are many amazing ways to prepare eggs. A restaurant may have a special way of preparing eggs that you may have never tried before. Always go for the egg dishes.

- » **Meats:** Look for fatty meats like pork belly or a nice ribeye steak. Always choose chicken thighs over chicken breasts.

- » **Seafood:** Fish with the skin on gives you some healthy fats and some beneficial omega-3 fatty acids.

- » **Veggies:** Look for your favorite low-carb veggies and remember that some veggies (like peas and corn) are high in carbs and should be avoided. Not all veggies are good for the keto dieter! Don't despair; there are plenty of low-carb vegetables that you can order. For example, broccoli, cauliflower, asparagus, and zucchini are all low-carb.

Looking at online menus before you arrive

More and more restaurants are adding low-carb options to their menus as well. This helps take the guesswork out of ordering even more!

It's always a good idea to look at a restaurant's menu online before you reserve a table. You can assess the menu in the comfort of your own home without feeling rushed or pressured to order. See what catches your eye and then dig a little deeper into that menu item. Some restaurants list ingredients of the foods as well, which is very beneficial. You may even get lucky enough to have a nutritional label attached to each menu item. This is the keto jackpot! It really gives you the chance to see whether the foods that you want to order are okay on your diet.

Reading the menu online also gives you a chance to see whether the food at the restaurant meets any other dietary concerns you may have. If you need a gluten-free dish or a restaurant that is nut-free, their website may help you find these specific details.

REMEMBER

Restaurants often run specials that may fit into your keto diet as well. These specials are likely not listed on the website, but you can call and ask about them in advance. You can also ask about the kitchen's ability to accommodate special requests. Speaking to a real person can be very helpful.

Tips and tricks for salad dressings

Salad is usually a safe keto order. You can't go wrong with lettuce and low-carb veggies. You do, however, want to be wary of certain salad dressings. They can be a source of many hidden carbs. Here are a few tips to ensure you don't get in the carb-loaded salad dressing trap:

>> Creamy dressings are just as good as oily dressings. They are often made with mayonnaise or yogurt, two delicious keto ingredients. Ranch dressing and blue cheese dressing are two very strong tasting, delicious options. You can use these dressings not only on salad, but as a dip as well.

>> Italian dressing is usually made with olive oil, lemon juice, herbs, and seasonings. It is a dependable dressing choice.

>> Skip any dressing with balsamic vinegar. Balsamic vinegar is high in carbs even though it is a vinegar. It is quite sugary and may kick you out of ketosis.

REMEMBER

Salad dressing can be a source of hidden carbs due to added sugar. Ask your server what brand of salad dressing they use and try looking up the nutrition label on your phone. If the dressings are homemade, the chef should be able to tell you the ingredients. A little olive oil, white vinegar, salt, and pepper is a simple dressing substitute that most restaurants are able to serve. All the fresh veggies, protein, and healthy fats in your salad should be flavorful enough that you can even just use pure olive oil.

Making Special Requests

Restaurants are very used to people asking for foods to be prepared in special ways. Keep this in mind and never be afraid to ask for small menu tweaks to get a food you can enjoy without worry. You should never get stuck ordering carb-loaded foods; there's always a way to reduce or eliminate the carbs! Servers and kitchen staff are trained to accommodate simple requests you may have. That said, try to be respectful of their carefully curated menu. Changing up too much of the original dish may be seen as unreasonable. The server will have no problem skipping your table's breadbasket though!

The more you eat out while on a keto diet, the more tricks you discover. You quickly figure out what substitutions are doable and which ones you prefer. You also get more used to asking for what you want.

Here are a few common customizations that benefit any keto dieter. Keep these tips in mind the next time you go out, and you can be sure to have a fantastic, keto-approved meal.

Replace starches with veggies

One of the easiest menu switches is to ask your server to replace any starchy side dishes with vegetables. Things like potatoes, sweet potato fries, or pasta can be replaced with a side of garlicky steamed spinach, a roasted veggie medley, or a tasty kale salad.

Look at what veggies are on the restaurant menu and use those as a guide to tell you what the kitchen should be able to make. Any vegetable side dish should be able to replace a starch side dish.

REMEMBER

Some restaurants may charge you for extreme substitutions. While spinach may be considered an equal replacement for mashed potatoes, a special kale and blue cheese salad as a substitute may cost a little extra. It may cost more in ingredients, and the chefs may need to take time to prepare your special food. Keep this in mind so the bill doesn't come as a surprise.

Choose butter, cream or a high-fat sauce and skip the gravy

When it comes to gravy, you want to steer clear. While gravy is high in fat, it's also almost always thickened with flour or another starch. If you are worried about other sauces on the restaurant menu, you can always play it safe and just ask for a side of melted butter. It can add enough richness and flavor to keep your taste-buds satisfied.

You can also replace a lower-fat sauce with a heavier one to increase your fat intake. Being able to freely enjoy fatty, creamy sauce is one of the benefits of keto. Look at the restaurant menu and see what types of sauces they serve. You should be able to choose the entrée you want with any sauce that the restaurant serves. Here are a few of our favorites:

>> **Hollandaise sauce:** This is a classic sauce made with egg yolks, melted butter, and lemon juice. It's often served with eggs benedict, but it goes with so many other foods as well. Add hollandaise sauce to your steamed veggies, fish, or even your favorite chicken dish.

>> **Alfredo sauce:** Alfredo sauce is made with cream, Parmesan cheese, garlic, and a little salt and pepper. It's usually served on pasta, but it's delicious poured over a nice juicy steak.

>> **Buffalo sauce:** Buffalo sauce may not be a cream sauce, but it is surprisingly good for keto dieters, so we had to include it on our list. Buffalo sauce is usually made with butter, so it not only adds spicy flavor to your meal, but it also increases the fats.

>> **Béarnaise sauce:** This creamy, thick sauce is like hollandaise, but it has a little bit of a spice to it. It is great as a steak sauce or as a dipping sauce for veggies.

REMEMBER

Don't be afraid to ask your server what ingredients are used to make a sauce. Every restaurant is different, so you may be surprised by what sauces are high in carbs.

Chain restaurants often have their ingredient lists and nutritional facts online. Do your research before dining out and you may be able to find very specific info about the foods on the menu.

Request a lettuce wrap instead of a bun or sandwich bread

One of our favorite substitutes for bread is lettuce. Almost every restaurant has a big piece of lettuce they can use to wrap up your burger or sandwich. It's a very easy switch.

We love using lettuce in place of a burger bun or bread because it allows you to still eat the food with your hands. When you skip the bun, you often end up eating the burger with a fork, which just doesn't have the same appeal. When you wrap the burger in lettuce, you can pick it up to eat and even enjoy the crunch of the lettuce along with the juicy burger. A big piece of lettuce should be able to hold condiments or burger toppings.

Ask your server to wrap sandwich fillings inside a piece of lettuce. If they are unsure how to do this, just ask for the lettuce on the side and you can wrap it all up yourself!

REMEMBER

Large romaine leaves are best for making wraps. The leaves are soft and tender, so they are flexible enough to roll. We like buttercrunch lettuce when it comes to burgers. A big piece of buttercrunch on top and one on the bottom make a perfect burger "bun."

Ask for extra fats

One way to ensure that you meet your keto diet fat needs is to ask for extra fats to be added to your meals. There are very simple ways to do this. Here are a few tips to help boost the fat content of your restaurant meal, ensuring you meet your keto macro requirements:

>> **Ask for extra cheese.** Request more blue cheese in your salad or for some extra Parmesan cheese to be melted over your steak. Cheese is a keto dieter's friend. Adding more cheese is something very simple that a restaurant can do to boost the keto appeal of your meal.

>> **Use more butter.** All restaurants have butter, ghee, or olive oil. Pour a little extra over your proteins, on your veggies, and into your salad. You'll be increasing the fat content and the flavor.

>> **Skip the sides and add more protein.** If the restaurant side dishes all look high in carbs, try asking for double the protein instead. The second serving of protein may be a little smaller (side dishes usually cost less than meats and seafood), but it will be keto-friendly and increase your protein and fat counts. You can ask for a surf-and-turf plate, giving you one serving of meat and one serving of seafood.

Opting for a Low-Sugar Beverage

Part of dining out is often not just the food, but also the wide array of drink choices a restaurant offers. This can be dangerous for a keto dieter. A tempting drink list may be trouble, but a trained keto dieter like you can choose wisely.

Water, of course, is always the best and safest choice. It keeps you hydrated and is guaranteed to have no carbs. Ask for a wedge of lemon or lime to make your water a little bit more flavorful.

If you want something more exciting, give one of these drinks a try:

>> **Sparkling water:** Adding a few bubbles to your water can make all the difference. Water is no longer boring when it's bubbly.

>> **Coffee:** An after-dinner mug of coffee is a great way to end a meal. Ask for your coffee black or add some pure heavy cream. Half-and-half is also a good option; just be sure to skip the sugar.

>> **Tea:** You can choose from any herbal, black, or green tea. Steer clear of fruit teas, which often have sugars mixed into the tea bags. Iced tea is also a safe bet if it's unsweetened.

>> **Dry wine or low-carb wine:** Most dry wines (whether red or white) tend to be the lowest carb choice among wines. Avoid sweet wines like dessert wine, Moscato, and port. You can also find more low-carb wines now on the market, which is very good news for keto dieters.

>> **Light beer:** Low-carb beer has even less sugar than wine. It's a good choice on the drink list, especially if you are out celebrating. Many beers are served in the bottle, so you can check the label and really keep track of the carbs you are drinking. Be sure to stick to just one beer because it still has carbs that can sneak up on you.

Dining at a Friend's House

Dining with your family and friends is an important part of life, but it often involves food prepared by someone who may not be aware of your new keto preferences. Communicate with them about your new diet and always offer to whip up a delicious keto option the whole group may enjoy as well.

At a party or a potluck, some type of protein or fat should always be served. Simply try to avoid any carbs that are served alongside them.

You may also be met with some weird looks if you decide to bring up the fact that you no longer eat carbs. Simply let others know a little about what you've discovered about the standard American diet versus your new diet choices, and say you're giving it your best shot.

These are a few clear and polite responses to the unavoidable keto nonbeliever comments:

» "Thank you, but I made a commitment recently to cut out high-carb foods for my health."

» "No thanks, I'm all set with [whatever high-carb food you're avoiding], but I'll take an extra serving of those greens or meat [or another low-carb food]."

» "That looks wonderful, but I'm really enjoying [a specific low-carb food on the table] at the moment."

One of the best ways to show people just how delicious it can be to eat keto is to bring their attention to a keto dish on the table. Perhaps it's one that you brought!

TIP

Don't be shy about sharing your new diet path. Your hosts would much rather know the reason why you're bringing specific food and avoiding others. An open line of communication is always better than secretly avoiding carbs all night.

Chapter 7

Maximizing Keto with Intermittent Fasting

ntermittent fasting is an eating pattern where you go through periods of eating and fasting. Intermittent fasting on its own is not really about your diet but more of a guideline for when to eat.

Intermittent fasting as a non-religious practice has been investigated as early as the 1910s for the treatment of obesity. In the 1940s, through lab experiments on animals (mostly mice), researchers discovered that by restricting calories, without malnutrition, through intermittent fasting, their test subjects' life spans had been extended.

In 2012, BBC journalist, Michael Mosley, popularized the 5:2 "diet," another form of intermittent fasting where you routinely eat five days of the week and greatly restrict your calories (around 500–600 per day) for two non-consecutive days of the week. The popularization of the 5:2 fasting method put intermittent fasting in the spotlight and set off a chain reaction of new studies and new methods being discovered and rediscovered, placing intermittent fasting front and center in the diet world.

In this chapter, we discuss the full range of benefits of intermittent fasting and a few of the methods you can try. Almost every version of intermittent fasting is beneficial, so choosing which method works well for you is best.

WARNING

As with any big changes to your diet, you should always consult your physician, especially if you have type 1 or type 2 diabetes. With intermittent fasting, even when consuming the same number of calories and grams of carbohydrates in the day, your blood glucose levels shift differently and can change your insulin dosing times and quantities.

Realizing the Benefits of Fasting

Intermittent fasting has many benefits, and scientists are discovering more and more each day. People have been practicing fasting for thousands of years. However, research is just now catching up to this method of eating and ceasing to eat to stay healthy.

Keto and fasting can go hand in hand beautifully. Intermittent fasting can help take your keto diet to the next level, ensuring your body is getting the most out of being in ketosis. Taking a break from food and letting your body reset naturally can be incredibly beneficial.

Accelerating fat loss

The keto diet helps your body become a fat-burning machine. Your body seeks out fats and uses them as fuel, but you may be surprised to discover that adding intermittent fasting to the keto diet helps speed up fat loss.

Normally, when you stop eating on a high-carb diet, your body automatically switches to burning fat after it runs out of glucose you've eaten or glycogen that's stored in your muscles. It no longer has a steady stream of glucose coming in the form of food. When you start fasting, your insulin sensitivity increases, and your body no longer wants to burn glucose and store fats.

With carbs out of the way, your body starts to burn fat rather than store it. Any fat that comes into your body is used to create energy, and if you need more energy, your body burns the fat stores in your body. You lose fat and are able to keep it off as your body no longer stores it.

Many changes in your body are from the "starvation" hormone called *adiponectin*. Adiponectin is boosted by fasting, and high levels of this hormone are associated with weight loss. People with low adiponectin levels are often found to struggle with insulin levels and type 2 diabetes. Some diabetes medications increase the levels of adiponectin in the body. The hormone is known to

>> Help you lose weight by lowering fat stores in your body

>> Reduce inflammation by stopping the release of fatty acids into the bloodstream

>> Lower your risk of diabetes and obesity

When you eat a keto diet, you are giving your body fats to burn. Your body naturally burns more fats from food before it switches to burning stored body fat. Fasting helps your body start going through all that stored fat. Intermittent fasting is a proven way to reach your weight loss goals by accentuating your keto diet.

Short-term fasting also helps increase your metabolism. Over the short term, the body's levels of adrenaline go up. While it is not healthy for your adrenaline to be elevated long term, it is very good as a short-term boost. Short-term adrenaline increases the release of excess glucose in your body. Getting rid of this glucose furthers your ability to burn fat. Studies have shown that your basal metabolism may increase by up to 12 percent during a short fast! This helps with weight loss quite significantly.

Enabling rapid muscle gain, repair, and recovery

Fasting not only helps you burn fat, but it can also help you gain muscle. This occurs in several different ways during a fast.

Improving muscle gain

The first way fasting helps muscle gain is by boosting the human growth hormone (HGH). This hormone is what causes development and growth in children and teens. HGH can

>> Increase muscle gain

>> Break down fats

>> Increase the growth of internal organs

>> Help improve bone strength and growth

>> Increase protein synthesis

Once you reach the end of your teenage years, this hormone naturally decreases and never really spikes again. Some adults take HGH shots to increase muscle mass and bone density and reduce fat. It is considered a doping agent in elite sports because it unnaturally improves athletic ability. HGH injections have harmful side effects like increasing blood sugar, heart problems, and possibly cancer.

Fasting provides natural bursts of HGH. You can get the muscle-building benefits from HGH through fasting, but you won't get any of the adverse side effects because it is being created by the body naturally.

Repairing cells to strengthen muscles

Another way that fasting helps increase muscle mass is by boosting the cell's ability to self-clean. Your cells are constantly working toward making your body clean and functioning properly. Cells identify any defects and repair you from the inside. They do this through two systems:

>> **Autophagy lysosome:** The process of "self-eating" where cells essentially destroy themselves as they get old, damaged, or overly stressed. The cell parts are recycled as energy.

>> **Ubiquitin proteasome:** The main system for breaking down short-term proteins within the cells. It is important to keep your immune system functioning and repairing your DNA.

If part of a cell becomes damaged, it needs to be repaired so the whole cell doesn't suffer. Damaged muscle cells can lead to feelings of weakness or even muscle degeneration. Muscle cells frequently need to be repaired because they are highly active, constantly bending and stretching throughout the day. Your body needs the tools and the proper systems to repair these cells to maintain muscle function and muscle mass.

Fasting helps improve the autophagy system and keep your cells healthy and functioning properly. Athletes have used intermittent fasting for decades to improve muscle health.

Helping muscles recover

Fasting can not only boost your muscle mass and repair your muscles, but it can also help your muscles recover. Fasting may

>> Reduce the oxidative damage to your body's protein

>> Decrease oxidative damage to DNA cells

>> Limit the buildup of dysfunctional cell proteins

Fasting affects your body's insulin levels and influences a hormone called *insulin-like growth factor 1* (IGF-1). IGF-1 can increase high blood sugar and has also been linked to certain cancers. Excess IGF-1 decreases the body's ability to manage and repair abnormal cells. People who have an IGF-1 deficiency have been shown to have extreme resistance to cancer. Many doctors even recommend fasting in conjunction with chemotherapy to reduce IGH-1 levels.

Levels of IGF-1 decrease in the body during a fast. This allows the body to find and repair more damaged cells that may have been missed when IGF-1 levels were too high. Intermittent fasting as part of the keto diet also helps decrease the levels of this harmful hormone and helps your body repair and recover cellular proteins.

Improving skin tone

Did you know that fasting can help improve your skin? We didn't know about this fantastic side effect either! Intermittent fasting combined with keto may impact the skin better than any face wash, toner, or topical medication combined.

Fasting helps improve your skin thanks to the significant amount of anti-inflammation that occurs when you fast. Inflammation and stress cause you to have breakouts and other skin issues. Fasting is a great way to relieve stress from the body, letting it take a break from processing all different kinds of food and using energy to recharge instead. Fasting allows the digestive system to take a break, increasing the billions of healthy bacteria in your gut. The anti-inflammation properties of keto not only results in nice-looking skin, but also gut health has been linked to skin health. The digestive system has the highest number of immune cells within the whole body. A healthy, clean gut has an increased number of immune cells and boosts your overall immunity. Higher immunity means your body can fight blackheads and acne, and even reduce small wrinkles.

Here are a few findings from recent studies regarding fasting and skin care:

>> Intermittent fasting helped improve wound healing in mice. It also improved the thickness of the mice's fur by increasing blood flow to the skin.

>> Fasting can work in conjunction with your regular skincare regimen. Fasting while using a topical retinoid may decrease the side effects of the retinoid, helping the skin stay hydrated and less irritated by the retinol.

>> Fasting lowers inflammation, which can help improve skin conditions like psoriasis and eczema.

>> Fasting reduces sebum, an oil that can clog pores and cause acne. Sebum was reduced up to 40 percent in some studies, which greatly helped prevent future acne and breakouts.

Another key to fasting and great skin is hydration. Remember to drink plenty of water. Water is the best thing to drink on a keto diet and during a fast, so drink up!

Slowing aging

Fasting has been shown to help you live longer. Allowing your body to fast improves its ability to heal and recover from certain diseases and infections. When your body can fully recover and heal, it is healthier in the long run.

Insulin and glucose both decrease significantly when you fast. Both are strongly linked to disease and rapid aging. Fasting for a full three days can drop insulin and glucose levels by up to 30 percent.

Fasting also decreases IGF-1, a hormone that is linked to certain types of cancers (see the earlier section "Helping muscles recover"). Fasting has been shown to reduce IGF-1 by up to 60 percent. These decreases improve longevity and contribute to long-term, overall health.

Scientists have found that the telomere part of the chromosome may be essential to preventing aging. The *telomere* is like a cap at the end of the chromosome. It protects the chromosome from unraveling and falling apart. As you age, your telomeres get shorter and smaller, which means chromosomes are more likely to be damaged as they no longer have the protection they once did. This is one reason why scientists believe older people are more susceptible to disease, infections, and cancers. The chromosomes are more at risk.

Studies have shown that long-term fasting can help increase autophagy, and autophagy is known to help elongate telomeres. This means that fasting can help prevent aging, boost your cells' ability to promote autophagy, increase the telomere cap on your chromosomes, and live a longer, healthier life.

While short-term fasting has many benefits, long-term fasting boosts autophagy. A prolonged fast of three full days or more is recommended to get the full effects of autophagy. You may need to work your way up to a fast of this magnitude and possibly consult your doctor or nutritionist first. The benefits of a long fast are great, but you still want to be sure you fast in a safe, healthy way.

Improving brain function

Fasting can seem intimidating, and many have concerns regarding fasting while still performing day-to-day tasks. Will you have enough energy to get through the day without any food? The answer is yes. Many people report feeling sharper and more alert when fasting. Mental clarity will improve as you go through a fast. When your stomach is full, much of your energy goes toward digesting food.

Fasting often and long-term fasting never affect the size of your brain. While other muscles may deteriorate if you fast for weeks at a time, the brain always stays the same size. This is because your brain is your body's biggest asset. We have evolved as a species to protect our brains. Outsmarting a predator is the only way to survive; we need our brains to stay sharp even when hungry.

The brain does need some glucose to survive. However, if you are not consuming any foods, your body can use gluconeogenesis to convert fatty lipids into glucose, feeding the brain despite having no new glucose sources available. You can survive up to 30 days without food as your system will prioritize nutrients to the brain.

Fasting directly affects the growth and function of neurons in the brain and brain cells. Calorie restriction and fasting increase neuron activity inside the hippocampus. This helps the brain in several ways:

>> By growing and maintaining the neurons' receptors, making them more able to receive messages from your body

>> By growing and maintaining synapses, the space between neurons necessary for communication throughout the brain

>> By allowing growth of brain stem cells and more neurons

Studies have been performed on rats that show intermittent fasting improves their ability to run through a maze and complete other memory-related activities. Further research is being done on the effects of fasting on Alzheimer's disease, which attacks the hippocampus, leading to memory loss. The results are positive as more and more ways that fasting can help with cognitive function are discovered.

Reducing inflammation

Inflammation is one of the leading causes of modern disease. From cancer to heart disease, many debilitating health issues can be traced back to inflammation. Nutritionists are constantly searching for anti-inflammatory diets to help prolong life and prevent deteriorating health. They find, time and again, that fasting is often the best anti-inflammatory diet out there.

We have already discussed type 2 diabetes and how it is caused primarily by inflammation and reduced insulin sensitivity. Here are a few other diseases that are triggered by inflammation:

>> Obesity

>> High blood sugar

>> High triglycerides

>> Cholesterol issues

>> High blood pressure

Fasting has been shown to help improve all these diseases, with alternated day fasting being the most beneficial. Those who cut their calorie intake drastically every other day found their blood pressure lower, increased weight loss, and improved insulin sensitivity.

The driver behind anti-inflammation is the fasting effect on *Sirtuin 1* (SIRT1), an enzyme that blocks inflammation throughout your system. SIRT1 turns off the genes that increase stress-related inflammation in your body (also a possible trigger for cancer). It helps to stabilize proteins in your body and help them function longer, allowing your body to maintain cells while reducing waste.

Adiponectin, the starvation hormone, is also boosted during fasting. This hormone is also an anti-inflammatory and may help reverse early stages of heart disease. Raised levels of adiponectin lower the levels of plaque inside the arteries. Some studies have shown that adiponectin may also help protect the liver from damage.

Detoxifying cells

Periods of detoxification are highly beneficial to the body. Your systems need time to clear out any damaged cells. When the body goes through the process of autophagy, the lysosomes within the cell search for any damage or abnormalities within the cell. Lysosomes then repair that damage or destroy the cell. This is the body's way of continually renewing itself.

Autophagy is an essential part of maintaining the body, but this process is often blocked by

>> High levels of insulin

>> Too much glucose

>> Difficult proteins

Even on a keto diet, fasting can increase all these things, making autophagy challenging. Autophagy can easily occur during fasting when no foods are processed and molecules don't get in the way.

Autophagy has been shown to be imperative in

>> Cellular survival

>> Organ maintenance

>> Controlling metabolism

>> Preventing cancer

>> Boosting immunity

>> Inflammation management

Autophagy has even been shown to help decrease the possibility of Alzheimer's disease. It destroys an abnormal protein called *amyloid beta*, a protein in the brain cells that can cause memory issues. Autophagy removes amyloid beta and prevents it from accumulating and causing early onset Alzheimer's disease.

Fasting allows your body to go through autophagy freely, cleaning out your cells in the most efficient way. It can also minimize the effects of stroke, brain injury, seizures, and even spinal cord injuries. There are far more benefits to fasting than to snacking.

Choosing a Fasting Method

There are many different ways of fasting, and choosing the one that fits your lifestyle is essential. You can benefit from each method; however, research has found that a minimum of 16 hours between meals is necessary to get the full effects of reduced inflammation and autophagy.

Here are a few different methods of intermittent fasting:

>> **Time-restricted eating:** You have set fasting and eating times in this option. Typically, people fast for 16 hours and eat for 8. Fasting for 18 and eating for 6 is also common but more difficult. Many people choose to schedule the fasting time while they are asleep so it's easier to stick to the schedule.

>> **5:2 method:** Eat regularly for five days a week and fast for two. This approach usually includes very small, 200-calorie meals on the fasting days. The idea here is to reset your system every few days.

>> **Alternate-day fasting:** This involves modified fasting every other day. On fasting days, you can still consume around 500 calories of high-fat, high-protein foods.

> **>> 24-hour fast:** This involves completely fasting for 24 hours. This is usually done once a week to reset your system, and then you return to your diet.

Essentially, you'll choose between a time-restricted fasting schedule or an alternate-day fast. Time-restricted fasts have you eat during a set time and then fast during the rest of the day. Alternate-day fasting requires you to stop eating altogether for 24 hours every other day. Many people choose a "modified fast" where calories are strictly reduced on the "fasting day," allowing around 25 percent of their regular caloric intake.

Common intermittent-fasting timelines

One of the most common fasts is the 16-hour fast. This method lets you follow your keto diet for eight hours during the day, eating all the healthy keto foods you like. Then, you fast for the remaining 16 hours of the day.

Since you can choose your fasting time, many people opt to fast from around 8 p.m. to 12 p.m. This fast is very doable for almost everyone. With this fast, your first meal is at lunchtime and should be the largest. It is also best to work out before eating that first big meal to help boost your metabolism.

Another option is the 18-hour fast. It's a bit more difficult than the 16-hour one, but people often start doing the 16-hour fast, get used to it, and then push themselves a little more to hit the 18-hour fast. Usually, the eating window is shortened by one hour on each end (for example, 1 p.m. to 7 p.m.).

Sticking to your preferred fasting schedule is essential. It makes it easier for you to maintain, and your body also benefits from anticipating when to fast and when to eat. Choose your schedule and plan your day around eating and fasting for the most success.

One meal a day

Another type of fasting you may want to consider is the 20-hour fast, also known as the "warrior diet." This fast gets its name from the Spartan warriors who would fast all day while fighting or exercising and then feast at night after the battle. This warrior approach is believed to help the body become lean and healthy.

The one-meal-a-day fast has not been studied as extensively as other diets, but since it is based on a time-restricted fasting method, it would seem to have the same benefits as the 16/8 method. A small study tracked people doing a 20-hour fast for six months. The participants experienced fat loss and muscle gain, but surprisingly, their blood pressure levels were increased.

During a 20-hour fast, you are allowed to eat a small number of calories outside your 4-hour eating window. It is recommended to time your eating period to the middle of the day and drop your calories by nighttime. Eating late can decrease your ability to sleep since your body is using energy to digest food.

Practicing a weekly 24-hour fast

Many people find the 24-hour fast the most appealing. You can fast once or twice during the week for a full day to give your body a complete reset. You also don't need to worry about tracking the time throughout the day when you dedicate a full day to fasting.

You can choose to modify a 24-hour fast a bit by eating between 500 and 600 calories. This isn't a true fast but more of an extreme caloric restriction, which can be a little easier to manage. The goal is to make a 24-hour fast part of your long-term way of eating, so you want it to be something you can do.

People who do 24-hour fasts say that hunger tends to decrease after they practice fasting for a few weeks. Many people find it liberating not to be bogged down by food and the need to eat. Be sure to check with your doctor before committing to a prolonged fast.

REMEMBER

Alternate-day fasting is similar to the 24-hour fast schedule but a little more intense. You fully fast every other day, dropping your calories to between 500 and 600 during your off days. While a 24-hour fast is good as a long-term plan, alternate-day fasting is best for the short term. It can help you lose weight quickly, boost your heart health, and lower triglycerides rapidly. Once you reach your health goals, you can try a once-a-week 24-hour fast to maintain your achievements.

Chapter **8**

Overcoming Obstacles

The keto diet is a fantastic one with such a long list of benefits. However, all those benefits only happen while you're in ketosis for extended periods of time (ideally for months or more). You'll want to know how to test for ketosis, especially initially. Eventually, once you've been in ketosis for a few months, you'll know if you're in ketosis by how you feel through your energy levels, mood, and other indicators.

Although there are tons of benefits with keto, it does have some drawbacks. There is no perfect diet out there, but the trick is to identify the obstacles and work toward overcoming them one at a time.

This chapter talks about some of the biggest keto obstacles, like initial side effects and social concerns, and helps you move past them. We have lots of tips to get you through some of the toughest moments in your keto diet.

Many of the issues people have with the keto diet are very short term. When you eliminate carbs and start eating high fats, it can be quite a big adjustment for your body. You may understandably encounter some changes and possible issues. Being prepared and planning ahead can help you greatly and that is what this chapter is all about.

Entered Ketosis and Staying There

We talk a lot about the body being in ketosis, but how do you know when you have entered this state? There are a few ways to find out whether you are in ketosis and truly on the path toward a successful keto diet. Once you know that you are in ketosis, you know that you are eating the right foods, balancing your macros, and off to a good start. Knowing that you are in ketosis can build your confidence and make you feel good just knowing you are on the right track.

Your body enters ketosis about three days after you start following a strict keto diet. You can start testing for ketosis and get accurate results at the three-day mark. These prompt results help you know whether what you're doing is correct.

Testing for ketosis

There are three primary ways to test for ketosis from home:

>> Urinalysis testing

>> Blood testing

>> Breath analysis

All the testing methods are fairly accurate, so you can choose the one that's best for you. Here is a little bit of information about each method.

Urinalysis testing

Urinalysis test strips check for excess ketones in your urine. The test strips are available at some drugstores and health food stores, or you can order them online. The small, paper strips have a spongy pad at the end, which is passed through your urine. The pad will change color, typically from a light to dark purple, if you are in ketosis.

If you are testing for ketosis daily, try to do a urinalysis test around the same time of day, preferably in the morning when your ketone levels are the highest.

REMEMBER

Urinalysis testing is the most cost-effective way to determine if you are in ketosis. This can be especially beneficial when you first begin your keto diet and don't want to spend too much money while ensuring you've entered ketosis.

Blood testing

Ketone blood testing is one of the most accurate ways to measure ketosis. It is also a more costly method because you need both the blood ketone meter and the blood strips.

Keto blood testing requires you to prick your finger using a lancet pen, extracting a drop of blood. The meter reads the level of ketones in your blood and gives you a number, which you can compare to the legend provided with the meter. You instantly know whether you are in nutritional ketosis.

Breath analysis

Keto breathalyzers are very convenient but not always the most accurate. Breath ketone monitors measure the amount of acetone in your breath, a side effect of ketosis. When you are in ketosis, the acetone levels in your breath are higher.

You can check your breath as many times as you like using the same convenient breath analyzer. There is no need to purchase new test strips as the meter is completely digital and one unit. A breath analyzer is good for controlling ketosis and using long term to monitor your diet.

Maintaining ketosis

The best way to maintain ketosis is to stick to your macros. If you do this, your body won't get kicked out of ketosis and you'll never have to worry!

When you first start the keto diet, it can be very helpful to have tools that help you monitor your diet. There are many apps that can track your foods and calculate your daily carbs, fats, and proteins. Be diligent about entering everything you eat into the app to ensure it is accurate. Get into the habit of opening your app and logging your food every time you prepare a meal. Don't forget to count the cooking oil!

Use ketone testing strips, a ketone blood monitor, or an acetone breath meter to check your ketone levels every now and then. Check more frequently when you first start on your keto journey. Knowing you are consistently in ketosis puts your mind at ease.

When you test your ketone levels and find that you are in ketosis, take note of how your body feels. Discovering what you, personally, feel like when you are in ketosis is important. Once you know how your body operates when in ketosis, you will no longer need tests strips or apps. You'll just *know* that you are in ketosis. Of course, a quick test never hurts, just to be sure!

Getting back into ketosis quickly

Whether you ate a carb-filled snack by accident or decided to try out a modified keto diet, there are times when your body may fall out of ketosis. It's important to get back into ketosis quickly so you can continue your keto journey.

You can always return to being keto and wait a day or two to naturally get back into ketosis. However, if you really want to get back on track as soon as possible, there are a few options.

Exercise is one way to help speed up the process and get back into ketosis. Moderate to extreme exercise gets your system moving and burns the stored glucose in your body even faster. When you exercise, you need more energy and fuel. Your body goes searching for that fuel and uses any extra glucose it can find. Make sure to exercise for at least 45 minutes to an hour (depending on intensity).

Another way to get back into ketosis quickly is through fasting for 16 to 24 hours. Fasting helps your body burn any remaining glucose in your body faster. Fasting can be difficult because it takes a lot of discipline. You need to resist eating and stick to water, black coffee, or tea only. See Chapter 7 for more information on fasting.

How quickly you get back into ketosis depends on how much glucose is in your system. If you had one sugary drink, it may only take 12 to 24 hours to get back into ketosis by just being keto again. If you went on a complete carb binge, eating bagels, pasta, and a big slice of chocolate cake, you may need to reboot your system longer.

If you are unsure about fasting to get back into ketosis, you can simply switch back to a hard, solid keto diet. Stick to completely carb-free foods and track your macros closely. You may experience some of the keto-flu symptoms (which we discuss in the upcoming section) you had when you first started keto, but hopefully, you'll dodge them entirely or they will subside sooner as your body knows what to do this time around.

REMEMBER

Just like when you first started keto, it can take a few days to get back into ketosis. Fasting and exercise can help you get back into keto faster, but a keto diet alone works as well. The best idea, of course, is to not fall out of ketosis, but we understand it happens! It's important to monitor your ketone levels and adjust your diet as quickly as possible if your levels drop.

Countering Common Problems

Many people experience the same problems when starting a keto diet. From common carb cravings to the "keto flu," you can expect some issues. But when you know the dietary issues that are going to come up, you can prepare for them!

In this section, we talk about all the common keto problems and how to tackle them head on. Accept that you may have a few challenges in the keto diet and then you will be better equipped to move past them.

Carb cravings

When you first begin on your keto journey, you may crave carb-heavy foods. This is completely natural since your body is so used to eating carbs. Stepping away from your normal eating habits is hard, and we understand this. Your body has been programmed to crave sugar.

Make sure you have some sweet and salty keto snacks available for when your carb cravings hit. Having something convenient and tasty on hand can help stop a carb craving in its tracks. There are plenty of keto-friendly baked goods you can make that are quite satisfying as well. You can still enjoy a nice piece of cake if it is a keto cake. Be prepared for the carb cravings, and you won't have to worry at all. Preparation is the key to success!

Increasing fiber intake

Fiber is an essential part of any diet. It is recommended that women under 50 get about 25 grams of fiber per day and that men under 50 get around 38 grams of fiber per day. Most Americans only eat around 15 grams of fiber a day, which is not nearly enough.

When thinking about fiber, keep in mind that there are two types of fiber:

>> **Soluble fiber:** Dissolves easily in water and can help reduce spikes in blood-sugar levels and improve cholesterol.

>> **Insoluble fiber:** Doesn't dissolve but attracts water into your stool, making it easier to pass. It also supports insulin sensitivity and helps promote bowel health and regularity.

It is important to get a good balance of both types of fiber in your diet. Soluble fiber, also called *prebiotics*, helps nourish the probiotic bacteria that live in your gut. Soluble fiber can convert to glucose if it is allowed to ferment in the gut. Therefore, many people used to add fiber to their daily carb count. However, many studies have shown that intestinal glucose lowers blood-sugar levels and helps the body get into ketosis. Fiber, on a keto diet, is a very good thing!

There are three things that fiber can do for you:

» **Slows sugar absorption:** Slowing the rate at which sugar enters your bloodstream can really help if you eat a few accidental carbs. If you have also been eating fiber, then you have a better chance of staying in ketosis. The fiber is like a sugar buffer.

» **Keeps you regular:** Fiber moves through your body faster than other foods, cleaning out your system and helping to regulate bowel movements.

» **Cleans your colon:** Because insoluble fiber can't be digested, it goes right into your intestines. It scrubs the sides of your intestines, cleaning out old bacteria and any buildup in your body. Not only does it keep you regular, but it also helps reduce your risk of colon cancers.

As you can see, you really want to be sure you are getting enough fiber while on a keto diet. So many health conditions can be solved by increasing fiber intake. Fiber also helps prevent hemorrhoids and diverticulitis. Now that you are likely to add more fiber to your diet, here are a few keto-approved foods that are high in fiber:

» Artichokes

» Asparagus

» Avocados

» Bell peppers

» Blackberries

» Broccoli

» Brussels sprouts

» Cauliflower

» Cucumber

» Garlic

» Green beans

» Lemons

» Limes

» Nuts

- » Olives
- » Onions
- » Radishes
- » Raspberries
- » Spinach
- » Strawberries
- » Tempeh
- » Tomatoes
- » Zucchini

REMEMBER

Fiber is like a "free" carb. You can always subtract the grams of fiber from the total carb count to arrive at net carbs.

Managing dietary restrictions

One of the biggest things that people worry about when considering a keto diet is the huge dietary restrictions. So many of us consume most of our calories in carbohydrates. If you are worried about finding good foods to eat, you are not alone. This is a concern many people have when looking at the keto diet, but the truth is, this couldn't be further from the truth.

A huge range of high-fat, low-carb foods is out there that you likely have not yet explored. Starting a keto diet opens an entire new world of foods that keeps you eating delicious, exciting foods. So put aside any worries you may have about keto being limiting and look at the recipes we've provided. We have so many great foods for you to try that you'll forget about carbs completely.

REMEMBER

Go into the keto diet with an open mind. Trying new foods is a fun part of the keto diet and it's something you should look forward to. Not only will you get to try new foods, but you *must* try new foods. Keto forces you out of your carb comfort zone, and we bet that you'll discover some new favorites along the way.

Dealing with Undesirable Side Effects

We want you to be excited about your new keto lifestyle but also be prepared for the downsides. All diets have potential negative side effects, but you should stay focused on the positive, long-term benefits of keto. Here are a few possible side effects that the keto diet may have and how to tackle them head on, making sure you are successful on your keto journey.

The "keto flu"

Many people talk about experiencing the keto flu when they start on a keto journey. Some, but not all, people experience flu-like symptoms when they stop eating carbs. It's not actually a flu and not contagious, but it can become quite tiring. Signs of the keto flu include:

>> Fatigue

>> Sniffles

>> Muscle aches and pain

>> Cough

>> Poor sleep quality

>> Brain fog

The symptoms mostly occur within the first few days or weeks of starting a keto diet. They can be rough! Your body needs to adjust to functioning with lower glucose levels and burning fats for energy. You also naturally lose water weight as you shed glycogen stores in your muscles. This loss of water can worsen the feelings of weakness and fatigue.

One of the main causes of keto flu is lack of *electrolytes*. Electrolytes are minerals in your body that carry an electric charge. Electrolytes affect the amount of water in your body, the acidity of your blood (pH), your muscle function, and other important processes. An electrolyte deficiency can be caused by a few things, most prevalent of which are your water intake and foods you may not be eating enough of.

Your potassium and magnesium levels may also drop, which is what causes those muscle aches. In addition, your body naturally misses sugar because sugar is quite addictive. There is a lot to get used to, but if you power through, you will come out on the other side perfectly fine!

You can completely avoid the keto flu by eating foods and drinking beverages that are high in electrolytes like

>> Chicken or beef broth

>> Unsweetened pickles or pickled foods

>> Generally salty foods or salting your meals more

If you start your keto diet eating these types of foods, you'll bypass the keto flu entirely or have extremely minor symptoms that will resolve in a day!

TIP

We have a few useful tips to help you survive the keto flu if you get it:

>> Make sure you are getting enough potassium and magnesium. Grab a few extra avocados or just try taking a multivitamin during your first days of keto dieting. These essential minerals help reduce your muscle cramps and make you feel less run down.

>> Drink chicken or beef broth or add a little salt to your water to ensure your body is getting enough salt.

>> Be sure to stay hydrated.

>> Rest! Allow your body to adjust to the new changes and rest as much as possible. Good sleep helps you transition much easier.

>> Pause your exercise routine. Give your body a break from hard workouts and don't sign up for a marathon. Let your body rest and adjust.

>> Ensure you are getting enough fiber to help your gut stay healthy and active.

The keto flu goes away quickly in the grand scheme of things. You will feel better in just a few short days. Your mood will improve right alongside your energy levels!

Cramps

Cramps, particularly in the legs, can occur when the minerals in your body are lacking or unbalanced, especially magnesium and potassium. When you are on a keto diet, your body loses water more rapidly and electrolytes tend to go along with it. Try to take a multivitamin or a magnesium supplement or increase your magnesium and potassium levels through your food intake to lessen your cramps. It's best to get vitamins and minerals from whole foods, but a vitamin can do in a pinch.

To help soothe cramps, try taking a bath in Epsom salts, getting a massage, or using heat therapy.

TIP

One ounce of almonds or ½ cup of spinach can provide you with 80 milligrams of magnesium. An avocado can provide 700 milligrams of potassium. Keep nutrient-rich foods in mind if you start having cramps when in ketosis.

Constipation

Many keto dieters experience constipation, which is often associated with losing water. Water exits your body faster when in ketosis, so you need to be sure you stay hydrated.

Fiber is also vital to help with passing bowel movements. Set a goal to eat around 25 to 30 grams of fiber a day. While fiber may be classified as a carb, it's a "free carb" because it passes right through your body mostly untouched. Nuts, seeds, avocado, vegetables, and berries can all help boost your fiber intake and keep you regular.

REMEMBER

To help remedy constipation, try the following tips:

>> **Drink extra water to ensure you are not dehydrated.** Water also lubricates your intestines and keeps things moving along smoothly.

>> **Exercise helps improve the flow of foods in your gut.** If you are feeling backed up, try going for a walk or an extra gym session to get things moving!

>> **Don't eat too much fiber.** Although fiber is critical for your diet, eating over 40 grams per day can cause constipation. Try to keep your fiber intake to 30 grams per day.

Diarrhea

While some people may suffer from constipation, others land on the opposite end of the spectrum and have a case of diarrhea. This is most common as you transition into ketosis and go through the keto flu. There are two easy ways to fix diarrhea caused by the keto diet:

>> **Reduce your intake of sugar alcohol sweeteners.** Eating a large amount of sugar alcohols can cause upset stomach and diarrhea. Reduce the amount of sweetener you use or try switching to a new brand. Maltitol is a cheap sweetener used by many big box brands when they create a sugar-free product, and it is known to cause diarrhea more than other sweeteners. Try a milder sweetener like erythritol or xylitol.

>> **Reduce your MCT consumption.** Many people use MCT oil to help get into ketosis but forget to lower the dose once they are on keto fully. Too much oil flushes out your system and causes diarrhea.

Diarrhea may also be caused by the increase in your dietary fats. It can take time for your body to adjust to a fat-based diet, so just be patient.

Keto breath

Many people notice that their breath smells sweet, fruity, and almost like acetone. Acetone, used often in nail polish remover, is a type of ketone, so this smell is perfectly justified. Some people even use keto breath testers to see if their body is in true ketosis by detecting the acetone.

This smell will go away after your body completely adjusts to the keto diet and reduces excess ketone production. Interestingly, some people never experience keto breath. However, if you feel like you have keto breath and want to get rid of it, here are a few things you can do:

» Increase your water intake to flush excess ketones out of your body.

» Practice good oral hygiene — brushing your teeth often and using mouthwash helps!

» Eat less protein. Protein is important on a low-carb diet, but when your body breaks down protein, it produces ammonia, which may be prevalent in your breath. Decreasing your protein intake may help improve your breath.

» Try carb-free gum or mints. Not only will they help your breath, but they can also curb cravings by keeping your mouth busy!

The biggest thing with keto breath is to be patient. It should go away as your body adjusts to the keto diet and starts effectively using all the ketones available.

REMEMBER

If your keto breath continues for more than a week, this may be a sign that you are eating too much protein. Excess protein can turn into ammonia, which you can smell through your breath. Double-check your macronutrients and consider making some adjustments.

Reduced strength or endurance

The keto diet ultimately gives you more energy than you have ever had before. However, you may find you experience a period of reduced strength and endurance at first. When you first stop eating carbs, your body may struggle to find energy. Once it learns to replace its carb-energy with fat-energy, you will gain back your strength.

Hair loss

The keto diet should not cause hair loss, but some people do start to experience loss of hair in the first few weeks. This is likely associated with the following:

>> Eating and drinking fewer calories per day

>> Vitamin and mineral deficiency

>> Low protein intake

>> High stress

When your body is fatigued, it uses all its energy to nourish your vital organs like your heart and lungs. The secondary areas, such as hair growth, suffer. This can be the cause of your hair loss. Be sure you are getting enough calories to give your body the energy it needs.

Check your protein intake and make sure you are getting the right quantity to succeed on your keto diet and keep your body strong. Also consider taking a multivitamin or finding ways to boost your B vitamins, which are important for energy metabolism.

Anytime you make a major life change, like starting a keto diet, you put stress on your body. Try to keep all the positive aspects of the diet in mind when battling any temporary side effects.

REMEMBER

Extreme hair loss can be caused by an underlying health issue. If your hair loss continues, consult your doctor to help discover the source. Keto, on its own, should not cause drastic hair loss.

Gallstones

Eating a high-fat diet, like keto, can help you flush out your gallbladder. In fact, if you already suffer from gallstones, increased fat intake can help push them out. If an existing gallstone gets stuck, you may suffer from gallbladder pain.

The gallbladder plays an important role in processing fats, so many people wonder if those who have had their gallbladder removed can still try a keto diet. The answer is yes! The gallbladder only stores bile, whereas it is your pancreas that makes the digestive enzymes to break down fats. The process may be a little slower, but your body, once again, will adjust.

Nutritional deficiencies

When you start a keto diet, you will likely switch the varieties of foods you are used to consuming. For example, people on keto tend to lose potassium naturally and may not be aware of keto-friendly potassium sources like avocados or cooked leafy greens. This can lead to a lack of certain vitamins and minerals. Some people feel the effects of missing nutrients in their diet. You may feel lethargic, run down, or even sick.

Taking a multivitamin to help you get the vitamins and minerals you need is a great option in the beginning. Fiber and MCT (medium-chain triglyceride) oil have also been proven helpful. However, once you build up to eating a wide range of keto foods, you should be able to get through this change. As you become better adjusted to the keto lifestyle and incorporate vitamin-rich, low-carb veggies, as well as a wide range of healthy whole foods, the need for a multivitamin will go away.

REMEMBER

Most new keto dieters don't have any nutritional deficiencies. It's entirely up to each individual to incorporate a wide variety of keto-friendly foods to ensure they get everything they need in their diet.

REMEMBER

KETOSIS VERSUS KETOACIDOSIS

Ketoacidosis should not be confused with ketosis — they are very different! Keto-acidosis occurs mainly in people with type 1 diabetes who can't produce enough insulin to keep up with the amount of sugar in the bloodstream. The body starts breaking down fat into ketones, but it does this while there is still excess sugar, which, if not processed, can be toxic. People who are in ketoacidosis have blood ketone levels of more than 25 mmol, whereas people in ketosis have levels that are less than 7 or 8 mmol. Ketoacidosis can lead to dehydration, vomiting, and belly pain, and you may even lose consciousness.

On a regular, maintained keto diet, you should never enter ketoacidosis.

Ketoacidosis most often happens in people who cannot process high blood-sugar levels. Healthy people who do not suffer from type 1 or type 2 diabetes should never experience this downside of the keto diet.

Alleviating Social Concerns

Drastically changing your lifestyle can be a daunting task. Your friends and family might be skeptical about your new life choice, but you need to keep your end goals in mind. Remember why you are choosing a keto lifestyle and all the positives that come along with it. While it may not be the path that most people choose, more people are starting to see the benefits. Be a leader and walk a path you can feel good about.

We have a few tips to help alleviate the social concerns you may have regarding the keto diet. Hopefully, reading them will help you stick to your decision and feel empowered by your choice.

Getting your doctor on board

More and more doctors are becoming well-versed in the keto diet as it gains popularity. However, many doctors are not fully aware of the numerous health benefits of keto. General practitioners do not always get full nutritional training in medical school, so your doctor may not be the best guide.

It's important to include your doctor in your keto journey, especially if you have pre-existing conditions and take blood-glucose stabilization medicine like insulin. Your doctor can assist you if you have specific questions about how the body works or if you are suffering from any side effects. Your doctor may take your cue and start brushing up on their keto education as well! Help get your doctor on board by sharing some of your keto research and keep them updated on your journey. You never know; you may turn your doctor into a keto believer.

Using your friends and family as cheerleaders

Your friends and family should want what is best for you. They should be the ones in your life who help you reach your goals and support your personal decisions. While they may not fully understand your new keto lifestyle, they should still be open to finding out about the benefits it offers.

Be sure to talk openly about your keto diet. Tell your friends and family about the positive impact it has and all the health benefits you can gain from a simple dietary change.

You are going to be the keto example for your friends and family. Teach them what eating a keto diet means. Tell them about the foods you can and cannot have.

Explain what keto means so no one is surprised or offended when you turn down that apple pie at Thanksgiving dinner. They may be genuinely curious and interested in the benefits for themselves.

Never be ashamed of your keto diet. It is not a fad but a diet choice with real, long-term, proven benefits. You are dieting for your health and wellness, not just to be "trendy."

Your friends and family can be helpful in your keto journey. They may be able to recommend delicious recipes or be a sounding board when you want to talk about the changes your body is going through. You don't have to go through keto alone! Even those who are not on the diet can help by cheering you on.

REMEMBER

Remember that the keto diet is your personal choice. While some of your friends and family members may want to try keto as well, don't force your dieting decisions onto others. Tell your family and friends about keto but don't expect them to change their lifestyle just because you did. Be respectful of others' dietary choices and, in turn, they should be respectful and supportive of your choice.

Planning for parties

If you are planning to attend a party or event, offer to bring some food! This is one of the best ways to show people how delicious eating a keto diet can be. You can prepare for a party by bringing a keto meal that you know everyone will love. Not only does this ensure that you have something safe to eat, but it may also surprise some nonbelievers. We have some incredible recipes in this book that are keto-approved and irresistible.

2

Creating Meals with Delicious Keto Recipes

IN THIS PART . . .

Get a strong start to your day with keto-friendly breakfasts.

Enjoy delicious keto appetizers with friends and family.

Savor warm low-carb soups.

Make quick-and-easy keto salads.

Prepare keto lunches to eat in or to take to work.

Try keto fish-based dinners for some variety.

Kick it up a notch with amazing meat-based dinners.

Chapter 9

Breakfasts

It is essential that you start the day with a good breakfast. The first thing you eat can really affect how you feel the rest of the day. Loading up on carbs will make you feel tired and even a little lazy. You need to break your all-night fast with foods that have some high-quality nutritional value and plenty of fat.

So many keto dieters turn to eggs as their go-to breakfast. We absolutely love eggs, but we also know that you may want something different and a little more exciting. We have plenty of tasty, creative egg recipes in this chapter, but we also go beyond the everyday egg.

You may be surprised to find how many sweet breakfast recipes we have created. We have keto-approved pancakes, waffles, and even tasty pudding that anyone who loves a sweet start to their day will appreciate. These recipes are just so good, you may even forget you are on a keto diet.

The keto life begins from the moment you wake up, so be sure to wake up in a good way with a delicious, healthy, low-carb breakfast. You will have more energy, feel fuller longer, and be generally happier after enjoying a delicious keto morning meal.

Porcini Baked Frittata

| PREP TIME: 15 MIN | COOK TIME: 30 MIN | YIELD: 4 SERVINGS |

INGREDIENTS

1 tablespoon olive oil

2 cups sliced porcini mushrooms

8 large eggs

¼ cup sour cream

Salt and pepper

½ cup chopped scallions

1 cup baby spinach, lightly packed

½ cup grated Parmesan cheese

DIRECTIONS

1 Preheat the oven to 400 degrees.

2 Add the olive oil to a large, cast-iron skillet and heat over medium-high heat.

3 Add the porcini mushrooms to the skillet and sauté for about 10 minutes or until all the liquid from the mushrooms has evaporated.

4 While the mushrooms cook, whisk together the eggs, sour cream, a sprinkle of salt and pepper, scallions, spinach, and Parmesan cheese.

5 Add the mushrooms to the egg mixture. Spray the skillet that was used for the mushrooms with a nonstick oil.

6 Pour the egg and mushroom mixture into the skillet.

7 Place the skillet into the oven and bake the frittata for about 20 minutes or until the eggs are completely set.

8 Remove the skillet from the oven, slice, and enjoy while hot.

PER SERVING: *Calories 234; Fat 17g; Cholesterol 338mg; Sodium 284mg; Carbohydrate 4g (Dietary Fiber 1g, Sugar Alcohol 0g); Net Carbohydrate 3g; Protein 16g.*

Avocado Omelet

INGREDIENTS

2 cups baby kale, washed and chopped

2 tablespoons olive oil, divided

½ cup cherry tomatoes, quartered

2 teaspoons balsamic vinegar

4 large eggs

¼ cup heavy cream

Salt and pepper

½ cup cheddar cheese

1 large avocado, peeled, pitted, and sliced

DIRECTIONS

1 In a bowl, toss the kale, 1 tablespoon of olive oil, tomatoes, and balsamic vinegar together. Divide the side salad between two plates.

2 In a small bowl, whisk together the eggs, heavy cream, and a sprinkle of salt and pepper.

3 Add the remaining tablespoon of olive oil to a skillet and heat over medium–low heat.

4 Pour the egg mixture into the skillet, cover with a lid, and cook for 5 minutes without stirring to set the eggs.

5 Sprinkle the omelet with the cheddar cheese and fold it in half, enclosing the cheese in the omelet.

6 Remove the pan from the heat and let sit for 2 minutes to allow the cheese to melt.

7 Place the sliced avocado on top of the omelet and cut it in half, placing each half on the plates. Enjoy!

PER SERVING: *Calories 653; Fat 58g; Cholesterol 388mg; Sodium 341mg; Carbohydrate 17g (Dietary Fiber 9g, Sugar Alcohol 0g); Net Carbohydrate 8g; Protein 23g.*

Raspberry Chia Pudding

PREP TIME: 5 MIN	COOK TIME: NONE	YIELD: 2 SERVINGS

INGREDIENTS

¼ cup chia seeds

1 cup almond milk

2 teaspoons low-carb pancake syrup

½ teaspoon almond extract

½ cup raspberries

½ cup chopped almonds

DIRECTIONS

1 Place the chia seeds, almond milk, pancake syrup, and almond extract in a bowl and stir well.

2 Let the mixture sit for 30 minutes; then stir again to break up any clumps.

3 Cover the pudding and put it in the fridge overnight.

4 Scoop the cold pudding into two cups and garnish with the raspberries and chopped almonds.

PER SERVING: *Calories 312; Fat 22g; Cholesterol 0mg; Sodium 92mg; Carbohydrate 6g (Dietary Fiber 18g, Sugar Alcohol 1g); Net Carbohydrate 6g; Protein 11g.*

Asparagus Eggs Benedict

| PREP TIME: 10 MIN | COOK TIME: 10 MIN | YIELD: 2 SERVINGS |

INGREDIENTS

Hollandaise Sauce (see the following recipe)

1 tablespoon olive oil

4 slices Canadian bacon

⅓ pound asparagus

Salt and pepper to taste

1 tablespoon white vinegar

4 large eggs

DIRECTIONS

1 Start by making the Hollandaise Sauce (see the following recipe).

2 Heat the olive oil in a large skillet. Add the Canadian bacon and fry for about 2 to 3 minutes on each side, browning the edges of the bacon slightly. Remove the bacon and set it aside, while leaving the bacon grease in the skillet.

3 Add the asparagus to the same large skillet. Cover and cook for about 3 minutes or until the asparagus is bright green. Season with salt and pepper to taste.

4 Fill a large pot with water and add the vinegar. Bring the water to a simmer, not a boil. Crack the eggs into individual rame-kins and slowly slide the eggs into the simmering vinegar water.

5 Poach the eggs for about 3½ minutes; then gently remove them with a slotted spoon.

6 Divide the asparagus between two plates and top each pile of asparagus with two slices of Canadian bacon, two poached eggs, and a drizzle of Hollandaise Sauce (see the following recipe). Enjoy immediately!

Hollandaise Sauce

INGREDIENTS

1 large egg

1 teaspoon lemon juice

Salt

2 tablespoons salted butter, melted

⅛ teaspoon cayenne pepper

DIRECTIONS

1   Separate an egg and save only the egg yolk. You can discard the egg white or save it for another recipe.

2   Place the yolk, lemon juice, and a little salt in a small bowl and whisk for about 30 seconds.

3   As you're whisking, slowly stream in the melted butter and continue whisking until a thick, foamy sauce has formed. Add the cayenne and whisk a little more just to mix it in. Set aside.

PER SERVING: Calories 268; Fat 20g; Cholesterol 915mg; Sodium 1340mg; Carbohydrate 4g (Dietary Fiber 2g, Sugar Alcohol 0g); Net Carbohydrate 2g; Protein 18g.

Cranberry Nuts and Yogurt Bowl

PREP TIME: 10 MIN	COOK TIME: 3 MIN	YIELD: 2 SERVINGS

INGREDIENTS

½ cup fresh cranberries

2 tablespoons granular erythritol

1 teaspoon vanilla extract

1 cup plain Greek yogurt

¼ cup chopped almonds

¼ cup chopped walnuts

DIRECTIONS

1 Place the cranberries and erythritol in a small pot.

2 Add a splash of water (about 2 tablespoons) to the pot and bring the cranberries to a boil over medium heat. You can add an additional 2 tablespoons of water if it evaporates before the cranberries begin cooking. They will begin to pop and "explode" as they cook. Stir continuously and cook for 2 to 3 minutes; then remove the pot from the stovetop. Let cool completely.

3 Stir the vanilla into the yogurt.

4 Add the cooled cranberries to the yogurt and stir only once or twice to swirl the yogurt and cranberries together.

5 Mix the nuts and place them in the bottom of two small bowls or cups.

6 Add the yogurt mixture over the top of the nut mixture. Garnish with the extra cranberries and serve.

PER SERVING: *Calories 305; Fat 23g; Cholesterol 19mg; Sodium 68mg; Carbohydrate 25g (Dietary Fiber 4g, Sugar Alcohol 12g); Net Carbohydrate 9g; Protein 15g.*

TIP: Make a big batch of the yogurt bowl ahead of time so you can quickly grab, eat, and go in the morning!

Sheet Pan Breakfast Bake

PREP TIME: 10 MIN	COOK TIME: 18 MIN	YIELD: 4 SERVINGS

INGREDIENTS

2 bell peppers, sliced (green and red work well)

1 medium zucchini, sliced

1 cup sliced red onion

1 pint cherry tomatoes, halved

2 tablespoons olive oil

2 teaspoons za'atar spice blend (or your favorite spice blend)

6 large eggs

DIRECTIONS

1 Preheat the oven to 400 degrees.

2 Place the sliced peppers, zucchini, onion, and tomatoes on a rimmed baking sheet.

3 Drizzle with the olive oil and sprinkle with the za'atar seasoning.

4 Bake the veggies in the oven for 10 minutes.

5 Remove the baking sheet from the oven. Stir the veggies on the sheet and then push the veggies aside to make small holes on the baking sheet. Spray each hole with nonstick oil.

6 Crack the six eggs carefully onto the baking sheet into the holes. Try to keep the yolks intact.

7 Return the baking sheet to the oven and bake for 6 more minutes for soft yolks, 8 minutes for firmer yolks. Serve hot.

PER SERVING: *Calories 137; Fat 9g; Cholesterol 240mg; Sodium 327mg; Carbohydrate 8g (Dietary Fiber 2g, Sugar Alcohol 0g); Net Carbohydrate 6g; Protein 7g.*

Bacon Egg Bites

INGREDIENTS

6 slices of turkey bacon

6 zucchini slices, about ¼ inch thick

6 large eggs

Salt and pepper to taste

DIRECTIONS

1 Preheat the oven to 400 degrees.

2 Wrap one piece of turkey bacon around the inside edge of each cup of a muffin pan. This will create a bacon ring around each muffin cup.

3 Place a slice of zucchini in the bottom of each muffin cup to create the base of the bites.

4 Bake for 10 minutes to soften the zucchini and start to cook the bacon.

5 Crack one egg into the center of each muffin cup, on top of the zucchini and inside the bacon.

6 Bake for 10 minutes more or until the egg is set and the yolk is cooked to your desired consistency.

7 Run a small spatula around the edge of the bacon cup to help release the mini bite and pop it out of the muffin cup. Season with salt and pepper. Enjoy while hot.

PER SERVING: *Calories 109; Fat 8g; Cholesterol 167mg; Sodium 135mg; Carbohydrate 1g (Dietary Fiber 1g, Sugar Alcohol 0g); Net Carbohydrate 1g; Protein 7g.*

Sweet Cheesy Keto Waffles

PREP TIME: 2 MIN | COOK TIME: 15 MIN | YIELD: 4 WAFFLES

INGREDIENTS

4 large eggs

4 ounces cream cheese ½ cup

1⅓ cup almond flour

¼ cup powdered erythritol

2 teaspoons vanilla extract

1 teaspoon baking powder

½ cup shredded mozzarella cheese

½ teaspoon ground cinnamon (optional)

DIRECTIONS

1 Place all the ingredients in a blender and puree on high speed. Stop the blender as needed to ensure all the ingredients are well mixed and nothing is sticking to the bottom of the blender. Puree until the mixture is smooth and thick.

2 Preheat the waffle maker as the batter sits for at least 5 minutes.

3 Spray the waffle maker with cooking spray and then pour about ¼ to ½ cup of batter into the waffle maker. (You may need more or less batter depending on your specific waffle maker.)

4 Close the waffle maker and cook for about 4 to 5 minutes, until the waffles are golden brown.

5 Use a fork to pop the waffle out of the waffle maker and cool slightly.

6 Cook the remaining batter using the same steps.

PER SERVING: *Calories 416; Fat 35g; Cholesterol 198mg; Sodium 330mg; Carbohydrate 22g (Dietary Fiber 4g, Sugar Alcohol 12g); Net Carbohydrate 6g; Protein 18g.*

TIP: Enjoy with low-carb whipped cream or fresh fruit.

Keto Chocolate Berry Smoothie

INGREDIENTS

2 cups unsweetened coconut milk

¼ cup unsweetened cocoa powder

¼ cup almond butter

2 tablespoons powdered erythritol

½ cup frozen blueberries

10 fresh blueberries

2 tablespoons shredded coconut flakes

DIRECTIONS

1   Place the coconut milk, cocoa powder, almond butter, erythritol, and frozen blueberries in the blender and puree until smooth.

2   Pour the smoothie into two glasses and garnish each with five blueberries and 1 tablespoon coconut flakes. Enjoy cold.

PER SERVING: *Calories 311; Fat 27g; Cholesterol 0mg; Sodium 17mg; Carbohydrate 31g (Dietary Fiber 9g, Sugar Alcohol 12g); Net Carbohydrate 10g; Protein 8g.*

Cabbage, Spinach, and Egg Hash Browns

PREP TIME: 15 MIN	COOK TIME: 7 MIN	YIELD: 2 SERVINGS

INGREDIENTS

6 large eggs

3 tablespoons minced garlic

1 teaspoon paprika

6 cups finely shredded cabbage

1 cup chopped fresh baby spinach

½ white onion, chopped

2 tablespoons olive oil

½ teaspoon salt

¼ teaspoon ground black pepper

DIRECTIONS

1 In a large bowl, whisk together the eggs, garlic, and paprika.

2 Add the shredded cabbage, spinach, and onion and mix.

3 Heat the oil in a large skillet and scoop 2 tablespoons of the cabbage hash brown batter in per hashbrown.

4 Cook for 4 minutes; then flip and cook for another 3 minutes until browned.

5 Season with the salt and pepper and enjoy while hot.

TIP: Serve with sour cream, chopped chives, or your favorite keto dips.

PER SERVING: *Calories 131; Fat 9g; Cholesterol 279mg; Sodium 113mg; Carbohydrate 7g (Dietary Fiber 2g, Sugar Alcohol 0g); Net Carbohydrate 5g; Protein 7g.*

Avocado Baked Eggs

PREP TIME: 5 MIN	COOK TIME: 15 MIN	YIELD: 2 SERVINGS

INGREDIENTS

1 large avocado, peeled, halved, and pitted

½ teaspoon sea salt

¼ teaspoon ground black pepper

2 large eggs

¼ cup chopped, cooked ham steak

1 tablespoon watercress sprouts

DIRECTIONS

1 Preheat the oven to 450 degrees and line a baking sheet pan with parchment paper.

2 Scoop out a tiny bit of the avocado flesh, making the hole where the pit was slightly larger in order to fit the egg.

3 Sprinkle the avocado with the salt and pepper.

4 Break each egg into a small bowl or ramekin and then slowly pour the egg into the avocado half, keeping the yolk whole.

5 Place the egg-filled avocados on an aluminum foil ring to keep them stable in the oven. Bake the egg-filled avocados for about 15 minutes or until the yolk has set.

6 Sprinkle the ham and watercress sprouts over the baked avocado egg and serve warm.

PER SERVING: *Calories 274; Fat 21g; Cholesterol 176mg; Sodium 364mg; Carbohydrate 10g (Dietary Fiber 7g, Sugar Alcohol 0g); Net Carbohydrate 4g; Protein 12g.*

Cheesy Egg and Sausage Breakfast Casserole

PREP TIME: 5 MIN	COOK TIME: 20 MIN	YIELD: 4 SERVINGS

INGREDIENTS

8 large eggs

¼ cup heavy cream

8 ounces shredded cheddar cheese, divided

1 pound breakfast sausage, cooked and drained

DIRECTIONS

1 Preheat the oven to 375 degrees. Grease a 9-x-13-inch baking dish with butter.

2 In a small bowl, whisk together the eggs, heavy cream, and half the cheddar cheese.

3 Pour the eggs into the prepared casserole dish.

4 Spread the sausage bits around the casserole dish evenly.

5 Sprinkle the remaining cheddar cheese over the eggs.

6 Bake the casserole for 20 minutes or until the eggs have set and the cheese is completely melted.

7 Slice and serve while hot.

PER SERVING: *Calories 651; Fat 47g; Cholesterol 491mg; Sodium 1626mg; Carbohydrate 4g (Dietary Fiber 0g, Sugar Alcohol 0g); Net Carbohydrate 4g; Protein 52g.*

Keto Yogurt Berry Bowl

PREP TIME: 5 MIN	COOK TIME: NONE	YIELD: 2 SERVINGS

INGREDIENTS

3 cups unsweetened whole-milk plain yogurt

1 tablespoon powdered erythritol

10 fresh raspberries

6 fresh blackberries

½ cup fresh blueberries

1 tablespoon hemp seeds

1 tablespoon chia seeds

¼ cup unsweetened coconut flakes

DIRECTIONS

1   In a small bowl, mix the yogurt and powdered erythritol. Divide the yogurt between two bowls.

2   Top each bowl with the raspberries, blackberries, blueberries, hemp seeds, chia seeds, and coconut flakes.

3   Serve cold.

PER SERVING: *Calories 329; Fat 20g; Cholesterol 31mg; Sodium 115mg; Carbohydrate 31g (Dietary Fiber 8g, Sugar Alcohol 6g); Net Carbohydrate 18g; Protein 15g.*

Cottage Cheese Pancakes

PREP TIME: 5 MIN	COOK TIME: 15 MIN	YIELD: 2 SERVINGS

INGREDIENTS

2 large eggs

½ cup whole-milk cottage cheese

1 teaspoon vanilla extract

1 tablespoon powdered erythritol

3 tablespoons coconut flour

¼ teaspoon baking soda

¼ teaspoon ground cinnamon

DIRECTIONS

1 Place the eggs, cottage cheese, vanilla, and erythritol in a large bowl and whisk together.

2 Add the remaining ingredients and whisk into a nice batter.

3 Heat a large skillet over medium heat. Grease the skillet with butter.

4 Per each pancake, add 2 tablespoons of batter to the skillet. Cook for 4 minutes, flip, and cook for another 3 minutes. You may need to cook the pancakes in batches, re-greasing the skillet in between each batch.

5 Serve the pancakes warm.

PER SERVING: *Calories 331; Fat 8g; Cholesterol 168mg; Sodium 432mg; Carbohydrate 15g (Dietary Fiber 4g, Sugar Alcohol 6g); Net Carbohydrate 5g; Protein 13g.*

Chapter **10**

Appetizers

What's dinner without appetizers? They're the first thing you eat ahead of a big meal. You need appetizer recipes that will fill up that empty stomach and get everyone excited for the main course. If the appetizers are good, everyone will know that dinner will be fantastic.

You don't need carbs to make great appetizers. In fact, the carb-heavy appetizers are typically the ones that go unnoticed. Everyone raves about how good a guacamole is or how great the homemade salsa was, but no one remembers the chips that were served on the side of those dishes. That is why we eliminate the unnecessary carbs and focus on the flavor-packed appetizers that give you all the "wow" and none of the "blah."

Appetizers can also play another fun role at a party. They can help your friends and family try a variety of keto foods in a casual, small way. If you bring out a tray of incredible almond flour jalapeño poppers, your guests will be so delighted by the flavor that they will never know they are eating keto foods. Use appetizers as an example of how great keto food can be. People are more likely to try one small appetizer than willingly sit down for a full keto meal. But once they are hooked on the apps, they're sure to inquire about more keto foods you can make.

Serve an array of keto appetizers at your next dinner party or just make one tasty recipe to have before your meal at home with family. We have plenty of recipes here to keep you busy for quite a while. There are always more on our website at www.tasteaholics.com/recipes/quick-bites if you need even more app inspiration.

TIP

Appetizers are a great way to increase your macros if you are falling behind. Eating too little on the keto diet is quite common because you're just not super hungry a lot of the time. Eating enough calories is still important; you just do it in a high-fat, low-carb way. If you notice your calorie count is down, try making a tasty snack or keto appetizer to add a few hundred more calories. You don't need to prepare a full meal, just a little something extra to give you the energy and nutrients you need.

Crispy Cauliflower Bites

INGREDIENTS

4 cups cooking oil for deep frying

2 large eggs

2 tablespoons heavy cream

1 cup grated Parmesan cheese

1 cup almond flour

1 teaspoon Lawry's seasoning salt

1 pound cauliflower florets, cut into bite-sized pieces

DIRECTIONS

1 Pour about the cooking oil into a medium pot and heat over medium heat.

2 In a small bowl, whisk together the eggs and heavy cream.

3 In a separate bowl, stir the Parmesan, almond flour, and seasoning salt together.

4 Dip the cauliflower florets in the egg mixture and then coat them with the almond flour breading. Let sit for a few minutes, then place the coated cauliflower into the hot oil.

5 Fry the cauliflower for about 4 to 5 minutes or until golden brown. You will have to cook the cauliflower in batches. Remove the browned cauliflower from the oil and place on a paper towel to cool slightly. Enjoy as is or with your favorite keto dip!

PER SERVING: *Calories 329; Fat 23g; Cholesterol 110mg; Sodium 668mg; Carbohydrate 11g (Dietary Fiber 5g, Sugar Alcohol 0g); Net Carbohydrate 6g; Protein 19g.*

Avocado Deviled Eggs

PREP TIME: 20 MIN	COOK TIME: NONE	YIELD: 4 SERVINGS

INGREDIENTS

8 hard-boiled eggs

1 large avocado, peeled and pitted

2 tablespoons lemon juice

1 tablespoon mayonnaise

2 tablespoons chopped red onion

1 tablespoon fresh chopped parsley

1 tablespoon fresh chopped chives

Salt and pepper

DIRECTIONS

1 Cut the hard-boiled eggs in half and scoop out the firm yolk. Place the yolks in a large bowl and the eggs on a serving tray.

2 Add the avocado, lemon juice, mayo, red onion, parsley, chives, and a sprinkle of salt and pepper to the bowl with the egg yolks.

3 Use a fork to mix the ingredients until they are nice and creamy.

4 Scoop the mixture into the hollowed-out egg whites, overstuffing the egg white with the avocado filling. You can also use a piping bag fitted with a star tip to pipe the filling into the egg white.

5 Chill the deviled eggs until you are ready to serve them.

PER SERVING: *Calories 233; Fat 18g; Cholesterol 321mg; Sodium 147mg; Carbohydrate 6g (Dietary Fiber 4g, Sugar Alcohol 0g); Net Carbohydrate 2g; Protein 12g.*

Almond Flour Jalapeño Poppers

INGREDIENTS

6 ounces cream cheese, softened

1 cup shredded cheddar cheese

¼ cup chopped, cooked bacon

12 jalapeños, tops cut off and seeds scooped out

1 cup almond milk

1 large egg

2 cups almond flour

DIRECTIONS

1 Preheat the oven to 350 degrees and line a baking sheet with aluminum foil. Spray the foil with nonstick cooking spray.

2 In a small bowl, mix the cream cheese, cheddar cheese, and bacon.

3 Scoop the cheese mixture into each hollowed jalapeño. Be sure to push the cheese mix all the way into the pepper, getting the cream cheese all the way to the bottom of each pepper.

4 Place the milk and egg in a shallow bowl and whisk together.

5 Place the almond flour in a separate bowl.

6 Dip the stuffed peppers into the milk-and-eggs mixture and then into the almond flour, coating the pepper completely in the flour. Let sit for a few minutes and then dip all the peppers again in the flour to ensure a good coating.

7 Place the coated peppers onto the baking sheet and bake for 15 minutes until golden brown.

8 Serve immediately.

PER SERVING: *Calories 431; Fat 37g; Cholesterol 80mg; Sodium 310mg; Carbohydrate 11g (Dietary Fiber 5g, Sugar Alcohol 0g); Net Carbohydrate 6g; Protein 17g.*

Buffalo Chicken Celery Boats

INGREDIENTS

2 cups shredded rotisserie chicken

¼ cup mayonnaise

½ teaspoon garlic powder

Salt and pepper to taste

¼ cup buffalo wing sauce

8 celery sticks

1 tablespoon fresh chopped chives

DIRECTIONS

1 In a large bowl, mix the shredded chicken, mayonnaise, garlic powder, salt and pepper, and buffalo wing sauce.

2 Cut each celery stick in half and place the halved sticks on a platter or tray.

3 Scoop the chicken mixture into each celery stick.

4 Sprinkle the celery with the chopped chives and enjoy chilled.

PER SERVING: *Calories 249; Fat 17g; Cholesterol 91mg; Sodium 981mg; Carbohydrate 4g (Dietary Fiber 2g, Sugar Alcohol 0g); Net Carbohydrate 2g; Protein 19g.*

Creamy Spinach Dip

INGREDIENTS

½ cup sour cream

1 cup softened cream cheese

10 ounces frozen spinach, thawed and drained

½ cup shredded white cheddar cheese

½ cup Monterey Jack cheese

1 cup shredded Parmesan cheese

1 tablespoon fresh chopped garlic

Salt and pepper to taste

DIRECTIONS

1 Preheat the oven to 350 degrees and grease an 8-inch square cake pan.

2 In a large bowl, mix the sour cream and cream cheese together until smooth.

3 Add the remaining ingredients to the bowl and stir together.

4 Scoop the mixture into the prepared cake pan and bake for 10 minutes until the dip bubbles. Enjoy while hot.

PER SERVING: *Calories 405; Fat 33g; Cholesterol 96mg; Sodium 828mg; Carbohydrate 6g (Dietary Fiber 1g, Sugar Alcohol 0g); Net Carbohydrate 4g; Protein 22g.*

Bacon-Wrapped Little Smokies

PREP TIME: 15 MIN	COOK TIME: 30 MIN	YIELD: 8 SERVINGS

INGREDIENTS

1 pound little smokies (or any small, cooked sausage)

12 slices bacon, each cut into three smaller pieces

¾ cup brown sugar erythritol

¼ teaspoon cayenne pepper

DIRECTIONS

1 Preheat the oven to 350 degrees and line a baking sheet with aluminum foil. Spray the foil with nonstick cooking spray.

2 Pat the little smokies with a paper towel to dry.

3 Wrap each mini sausage in a one-third piece of bacon and secure the bacon with a toothpick.

4 In a small bowl, combine the brown sugar erythritol and the cayenne pepper.

5 Hold the toothpick of each sausage and dip them into the sweetener mix one by one, placing them on the baking sheet after they have been dipped.

6 Bake the smokies for 20 minutes. Flip the smokies and bake for an additional 10 minutes or until the bacon is completely browned. Enjoy hot!

PER SERVING: *Calories 250; Fat 22g; Cholesterol 101mg; Sodium 1352mg; Carbohydrate 20g (Dietary Fiber 0g, Sugar Alcohol 18g); Net Carbohydrate 2g; Protein 9g.*

Baked Spinach Balls

INGREDIENTS

6 cups fresh chopped baby spinach

3 large eggs

1 cup shredded cheddar cheese

2 teaspoons garlic powder

1 teaspoon sea salt

1 cup almond flour

1 tablespoon psyllium husk powder

DIRECTIONS

1 Preheat the oven to 350 degrees and grease a rimmed baking sheet.

2 Place the spinach in a large pan over medium heat. Using tongs, gently toss and turn the spinach so all of the unwilted leaves make contact with the bottom of the pan. If you can't fit all the spinach on the pan right away, you can add the rest after most of the spinach on the pan has wilted. When all the spinach is completely wilted and has turned bright green, it is done.

3 Remove the spinach from the pan and spread it out on a plate so the steam evaporates and it cools. Once the spinach has cooled, gather it into a ball and squeeze as hard as you can to drain any remaining water.

4 Place the dried, wilted spinach in a dry large bowl and add all the remaining ingredients. Stir to form a thick dough.

5 Scoop the dough into 1½ tablespoon–sized balls. You should get about 18 to 20 balls.

6 Place the spinach balls on a greased baking sheet and bake until golden brown, about 20 to 25 minutes. Serve while hot.

PER SERVING: *Calories 357; Fat 27g; Cholesterol 148mg; Sodium 264mg; Carbohydrate 13g (Dietary Fiber 7g, Sugar Alcohol 0g); Net Carbohydrate 6g; Protein 19g.*

Almond Halloumi Bites

PREP TIME: 10 MIN	COOK TIME: 12 MIN	YIELD: 4 SERVINGS

INGREDIENTS

2 tablespoons olive oil

½ pound halloumi cheese

½ cup almond flour

¼ teaspoon smoked paprika

½ teaspoon salt

1 large egg

DIRECTIONS

1   Preheat the oven to 350 degrees.

2   Line a sheet pan with aluminum foil and pour the olive oil onto the pan. Rub the oil all over to grease the foil well.

3   Slice the halloumi into 1-inch cubes.

4   In a medium-sized bowl, mix the almond flour, paprika, and salt together.

5   In a separate bowl, whisk the egg.

6   Dip the cheese cubes into the almond flour mixture and then into the whisked eggs. Once the cheese is coated in the egg, dip it back into the flour mixture and then place the coated cheese on the baking sheet.

7   Bake the halloumi cubes for 12 minutes or until golden brown, flipping them after 6 minutes. Enjoy while hot.

PER SERVING: *Calories 340; Fat 31g; Cholesterol 80mg; Sodium 617mg; Carbohydrate 3g (Dietary Fiber 1g, Sugar Alcohol 0g); Net Carbohydrate 1g; Protein 17g.*

Zucchini Chips

PREP TIME: 10 MIN	COOK TIME: 15 MIN	YIELD: 6 SERVINGS

INGREDIENTS

¼ cup olive oil

¼ teaspoon smoked paprika

½ teaspoon garlic powder

½ teaspoon salt

2 medium zucchinis, sliced into ¼-inch circles

¾ cup grated Parmesan cheese

¼ cup almond flour

DIRECTIONS

1 Preheat the oven to 375 degrees and spray two baking sheets with cooking spray.

2 In a medium-sized bowl, mix the olive oil, paprika, garlic powder, and salt.

3 Add the zucchini slices to the bowl and toss together, coating all the zucchini in the seasoned oil.

4 Line up the zucchini on the baking sheet in a single layer; do not overlap.

5 In a separate bowl, mix the Parmesan cheese and almond flour.

6 Sprinkle each zucchini slice with the Parmesan cheese mixture, covering each of the zucchini circles.

7 Bake the zucchini for 15 minutes. The tops of the chips should be golden brown. Bake for 5 more minutes if you want a crunchier chip.

8 Enjoy while warm.

PER SERVING: *Calories 159; Fat 14g; Cholesterol 15mg; Sodium 173mg; Carbohydrate 3g (Dietary Fiber 1g, Sugar Alcohol 0g); Net Carbohydrate 2g; Protein 6g.*

Zucchini Pizza Bites

| PREP TIME: 10 MIN | COOK TIME: 8 MIN | YIELD: 6 SERVINGS |

INGREDIENTS

2 medium zucchinis, sliced into ¼-inch-thick circles

½ cup Rao's tomato sauce

2 Roma tomatoes, sliced into ⅛-inch-thick circles

Salt and pepper to taste

1 cup shredded Parmesan cheese

Parsley or fresh basil (optional)

DIRECTIONS

1   Preheat the oven to 450 degrees and line a rimmed baking pan with aluminum foil. Spray with cooking spray.

2   Place the zucchini slices on the prepared baking sheet. It's okay if the slices touch.

3   Top each zucchini slice with about ½ tablespoon of tomato sauce.

4   Place a tomato slice on top of each zucchini.

5   Sprinkle the zucchini slices with salt and pepper to taste and then sprinkle them with the Parmesan cheese.

6   Bake for 8 minutes in the oven.

7   Garnish with parsley or basil, if desired, and serve while hot.

PER SERVING: *Calories 82; Fat 4g; Cholesterol 20mg; Sodium 315mg; Carbohydrate 3g (Dietary Fiber 1g, Sugar Alcohol 0g); Net Carbohydrate 3g; Protein 6g.*

Chapter **11**

Soups

A big bowl of warm soup can fill your belly and soothe your soul. Nothing is quite like that first, toasty sip. Homemade soups are especially delicious. You can tell when a soup has been made from scratch with love. A huge benefit of making soup from scratch is that you can alter the recipe, adjusting it to be exactly what you need. For example, you can make it completely low carb. That's exactly what we did with a few of our favorite soup recipes.

Soups are not typically low carb. Many soups have hidden carbs disguised as vegetables. Soups made with corn, potatoes, or lots of tomatoes may not be the best choice. Soups are often high in protein, which can be great on a keto diet if the protein in the soup fits into your daily macro count. Lots of soups have chicken broth or beef broth, which are both great for nutrients and vitamins. Don't be afraid to use some of the fattier cuts of meat for your soups. The extra fat is great for your keto diet and makes the broth taste smooth and silky.

Soup is perfect for lunch or dinner. It's a great way to soothe a sore throat or to help warm you up on a cold winter's day. With these soup recipes, you can enjoy every sip guilt free!

TIP

The best part about soups is they're all perfect for leftovers! You can keep just about any soup in the fridge for four or five days, reheating it when you are ready to enjoy it!

Bacon Butternut Soup

PREP TIME: 15 MIN | COOK TIME: 50 MIN | YIELD: 6 SERVINGS

INGREDIENTS

3 pounds chopped butternut squash

1 white onion, chopped

½ cup chopped red bell pepper

2 tablespoons olive oil

2 teaspoons minced garlic

Salt and pepper to taste

8 slices bacon, diced

3 cups chicken stock

DIRECTIONS

1 Preheat the oven to 400 degrees and lightly oil a rimmed baking sheet.

2 Place the squash, onion, bell pepper, olive oil, garlic, and a sprinkle of salt and pepper on the prepared baking sheet and toss everything together, coating the veggies in the oil.

3 Roast the veggies in the oven for about 25 to 30 minutes or until the squash is fork-tender. Remove from the oven and set aside.

4 Cook the chopped bacon in a large skillet over medium-high heat. Cook until the bacon begins to brown, about 10 minutes. Stir occasionally so the bacon cooks evenly.

5 Remove the bacon from the skillet and set aside.

6 Place the squash and roasted veggies in a large pot. Add the chicken broth and heat the soup to a simmer.

7 Use an immersion blender to puree the soup in the pot, blending until smooth.

8 Bring the thick soup to a boil and simmer for about 10 minutes; then stir in the cooked bacon pieces.

9 Scoop into bowls and enjoy!

PER SERVING: *Calories 224; Fat 11g; Cholesterol 12mg; Sodium 570mg; Carbohydrate 30g (Dietary Fiber 5g, Sugar Alcohol 0g); Net Carbohydrate 25g; Protein 5g.*

Italian Wedding Soup

PREP TIME: 15 MIN | COOK TIME: 25 MIN | YIELD: 8 SERVINGS

INGREDIENTS

Meatballs (see the following recipe)

12 cups chicken broth

1 tablespoon olive oil

¾ cup ¼-inch diced celery

1 cup ¼-inch diced carrots

6 cups baby spinach, lightly packed

2 teaspoons dried oregano

¼ teaspoon salt

¼ teaspoon black pepper

2 large eggs

DIRECTIONS

1 Start by making the meatballs for the soup (see the following recipe).

2 Pour the chicken broth into a large pot and bring to a simmer.

3 Heat the olive oil in a large pan over medium–high heat. Add the celery and carrots to the pan and sauté until the veggies have softened, about 6 to 8 minutes.

4 Add the celery, carrots, spinach, oregano, salt and pepper, and meatballs to the pot. Cook for 10 minutes.

5 Whisk the eggs in a bowl and slowly pour them into the soup, stirring as you pour.

6 Divide the soup among eight bowls and enjoy while warm.

Meatballs

INGREDIENTS

½ cup onion, diced

⅓ cup fresh chopped parsley

1 large egg

1 clove garlic, minced

1 teaspoon salt

½ teaspoon ground black pepper

¾ cup grated Parmesan cheese

½ pound ground beef

½ pound ground pork

DIRECTIONS

1 Place the onion, parsley, egg, garlic, salt and pepper in a large bowl and toss everything together.

2 Add the cheese, beef, and pork to the bowl and mix with your hands.

3 Use a tablespoon to scoop the mixture and roll it with your hands into small meatballs. Place the meatballs on a baking sheet and set them aside for use in soup.

PER SERVING: *Calories 237; Fat 16g; Cholesterol 115mg; Sodium 1546mg; Carbohydrate 5g (Dietary Fiber 1g, Sugar Alcohol 0g); Net Carbohydrate 4g; Protein 18g.*

Seafood Chowder

INGREDIENTS

4 tablespoons unsalted butter

1 tablespoon minced garlic

1½ cups chopped celery

1 cup clam juice

2 cups vegetable broth

1½ cups heavy cream

4 ounces cream cheese ½ cup, softened

2 teaspoons dried thyme

2 tablespoons lemon juice

1 pound tuna, cut into 1-inch pieces

½ pound shrimp, peeled and deveined

½ pound small bay scallops

½ teaspoon salt

½ teaspoon ground black pepper

DIRECTIONS

1 Place the butter in a large pot and melt over medium heat.

2 Add the garlic and celery to the pot and sauté for 5 minutes.

3 Add the clam juice, vegetable broth, heavy cream, cream cheese, thyme, and lemon juice to the pot and stir. Bring to a simmer.

4 Simmer the soup for about 5 minutes.

5 Add the tuna, shrimp, and scallops to the pot. Simmer for 5 minutes, stirring occasionally.

6 Add the salt and pepper, divide among four bowls, and enjoy.

PER SERVING: *Calories 752; Fat 56g; Cholesterol 318mg; Sodium 1020mg; Carbohydrate 9g (Dietary Fiber 1g, Sugar Alcohol 0g); Net Carbohydrate 8g; Protein 52g.*

Cream of Mushroom Soup

PREP TIME: 5 MIN | COOK TIME: 15 MIN | YIELD: 4 SERVINGS

INGREDIENTS

½ cup unsalted butter

3 cups sliced baby portobello mushrooms

2 cups sliced shiitake mushrooms

1 cup chopped white onion

4 cloves garlic, chopped

2 teaspoon dried thyme

4 cups chicken stock

1 cup heavy cream

½ teaspoon salt

¼ teaspoon ground black pepper

DIRECTIONS

1 Place the butter in a large pot and melt over medium-high heat.

2 Add the mushrooms and sauté until browned.

3 Remove about ½ cup of the mushrooms from the pot and set aside for a garnish.

4 Add the onion and garlic to the pot and stir. Sauté for another 3 minutes.

5 Add the thyme, chicken stock, heavy cream, salt and pepper to the pot and bring to a simmer. Simmer for 5 minutes.

6 Remove the pot from the stove and use an immersion blender to pulse the soup keeping small bits of mushroom intact.

7 Divide the soup among four bowls and top each with the reserved mushrooms. Enjoy while hot.

PER SERVING: *Calories 490; Fat 46g; Cholesterol 148mg; Sodium 1278mg; Carbohydrate 14g (Dietary Fiber 4g, Sugar Alcohol 0g); Net Carbohydrate 11g; Protein 8g.*

Sriracha Chicken Soup

PREP TIME: 10 MIN	COOK TIME: 1 HR AND 10 MIN	YIELD: 8 SERVINGS

INGREDIENTS

2 tablespoons olive oil

1 cup chopped white onion

1 cup chopped carrots

1 cup chopped celery

4 cups shredded, cooked chicken breast

10 cups chicken broth

1 tablespoon Italian seasoning

4 bay leaves

1 teaspoon salt

¼ teaspoon ground black pepper

2 tablespoons Sriracha

DIRECTIONS

1 Place the olive oil in a large pot and heat over medium–high heat.

2 Add the onion, carrots, and celery and sauté for 5 minutes, stirring occasionally.

3 Add the chicken and sauté for one more minute.

4 Add the chicken broth, Italian seasoning, bay leaves, salt and pepper, and bring to a simmer.

5 Cover and simmer for 1 hour, stirring occasionally.

6 Remove and discard the bay leaves.

7 Stir in the Sriracha; then divide the soup among eight bowls. Enjoy warm.

PER SERVING: *Calories 161; Fat 9g; Cholesterol 43mg; Sodium 1300mg; Carbohydrate 5g (Dietary Fiber 1g, Sugar Alcohol 0g); Net Carbohydrate 4g; Protein 14g.*

Creamy Broccoli Cheddar Soup

PREP TIME: 10 MIN	COOK TIME: 15 MIN	YIELD: 4 SERVINGS

INGREDIENTS

4 tablespoons unsalted butter

1 whole yellow onion, minced

1 clove garlic, minced

3 cups chicken broth

2 cups broccoli florets

½ teaspoon salt

½ teaspoon ground black pepper

1 tablespoon cream cheese, softened

¼ cup heavy cream

1 cup cheddar cheese

2 tablespoons sour cream

DIRECTIONS

1   Place the butter in a large pot and melt over medium-high heat.

2   Add the onion and garlic and sauté for 3 minutes.

3   Add the chicken broth, broccoli, salt and pepper to the pot. Bring to a simmer and cook for 5 minutes.

4   Use an immersion blender to pulse the soup keeping small bits of broccoli intact.

5   Add the cream cheese to the pot and stir to melt.

6   Add the heavy cream and cheddar cheese to the pot and stir to melt the cheese.

7   Divide among four bowls and top each with ½ tablespoon of sour cream. Enjoy while warm.

PER SERVING: *Calories 329; Fat 30g; Cholesterol 91mg; Sodium 914mg; Carbohydrate 8g (Dietary Fiber 2g, Sugar Alcohol 0g); Net Carbohydrate 6g; Protein 10g.*

Chapter **12**

Salads

When you think of diet food, you may automatically think of salads. Salads tend to be considered very healthy foods. All those leafy greens just look healthy. Most salads are nutritious, especially when they are carb-free.

The tricky thing about salads is that they can be low in fat. On a keto diet, you want the extra fats. You can add healthy fats to your salads in so many ways.

We like to make homemade dressings that are high in fat but still low in carbs. Lots of store-bought dressings have sugar added to the bottle. When you make your own dressing, you can use delicious extra-virgin olive oils, fresh herbs, and spices and get all the flavor you want without the carb overload.

Adding cheese and meats to salad is another fantastic way to boost the fat and protein count while still getting all the nutrients of a salad. Bacon, halloumi, Parmesan, and tuna are all so delicious. Enjoy a keto salad as a perfect lunch or even as a dinner. You can even have a small salad as a little snack. They are great for boosting your macros and helping you reach your targets in a tasty way.

TIP

Salads are typically best when made fresh. You can make a salad in advance and keep the dressing on the side until you are ready to eat. Dressing can make the lettuce soggy if left to sit too long. So, pack your salad in your lunch container, keep a little jar of dressing on the side, and drizzle it on when you are ready to eat!

Grilled Halloumi Salad

INGREDIENTS

6 ounces halloumi cheese, sliced-thick

1 ripe avocado, halved, peeled, and pitted

¼ cup olive oil, divided

2 garlic cloves, minced

2 tablespoons lemon juice

Salt and pepper to taste

4 cups baby spinach, lightly packed

10 grape tomatoes

DIRECTIONS

1   Preheat a grill pan over the stovetop or an outdoor grill to medium-high heat.

2   Brush the halloumi slices and avocado halves with 1 tablespoon of the olive oil.

3   Place the halloumi and avocado on the preheated grill and sear for about 2 to 3 minutes on each side or until grill marks appear.

4   While the cheese and avocado are grilling, make a lemon dressing by adding the remaining olive oil, garlic, lemon juice, and salt and pepper to a bowl and whisk until the dressing is very smooth and almost creamy.

5   Divide the spinach and tomatoes between two large bowls.

6   Slice the grilled avocado and divide it between the salad bowls. Top each with grilled halloumi and then drizzle with the lemon dressing. Enjoy while the cheese and avocado are warm.

PER SERVING: *Calories 526; Fat 48g; Cholesterol 12mg; Sodium 231mg; Carbohydrate 9g (Dietary Fiber 3g, Sugar Alcohol 0g); Net Carbohydrate 6g; Protein 23g.*

Basil Chicken Zoodle Salad

PREP TIME: 10 MIN | COOK TIME: 10 MIN | YIELD: 4 SERVINGS

INGREDIENTS

2 cups fresh basil

¼ cup plus 2 tablespoons olive oil, divided

¼ cup sliced almonds

1 cup grated Parmesan cheese

1 clove garlic

2 large boneless, skinless chicken breasts

3 medium zucchinis, ends trimmed

2 cups cherry tomatoes

DIRECTIONS

1 To make the pesto sauce, place the basil, ¼ cup of olive oil, almonds, Parmesan cheese, and garlic in a food processor and pulse. Set aside.

2 Add the remaining olive oil to a large skillet and heat over medium heat.

3 Slice the chicken breasts into smaller pieces, about ½-inch thick and 4 to 5 inches long.

4 Add the chicken breasts to the skillet and sear, cooking for about 4 minutes; then flipping and cooking for another 4 minutes.

5 Add half the pesto sauce to the skillet and toss the chicken to coat it with the sauce.

6 Cut the zucchini into long noodles (or zoodles) using a spiralizer, mandolin slicer, or peeler.

7 Place the zucchini zoodles in a large bowl with about 1 inch of water. Cover and steam in the microwave for 2 minutes.

8 Toss the steamed zoodles in the remaining pesto sauce.

9 Divide the zoodles among four bowls and top each with the basil chicken and the cherry tomatoes.

PER SERVING: *Calories 487; Fat 36g; Cholesterol 76mg; Sodium 292mg; Carbohydrate 6g (Dietary Fiber 3g, Sugar Alcohol 0g); Net Carbohydrate 6g; Protein 30g.*

Bacon Broccoli Salad

PREP TIME: 10 MIN	COOK TIME: NONE	YIELD: 4 SERVINGS

INGREDIENTS

⅔ cup mayonnaise

¼ cup apple cider vinegar

1 tablespoon mustard

Salt and pepper to taste

8 cups broccoli florets

½ cup shredded cheddar cheese

¼ cup chopped red onion

½ cup crumbled, cooked bacon

DIRECTIONS

1 In a small bowl, whisk together the mayonnaise, vinegar, mustard, and salt and pepper.

2 In a large bowl, toss the broccoli, cheddar cheese, red onion, and bacon together.

3 Add the dressing to the broccoli salad and mix well.

4 Divide among four bowls and serve chilled.

PER SERVING: *Calories 436; Fat 38g; Cholesterol 38mg; Sodium 551mg; Carbohydrate 14g (Dietary Fiber 5g, Sugar Alcohol 0g); Net Carbohydrate 9g; Protein 12g.*

Salmon and Kale Salad

PREP TIME: 10 MIN	COOK TIME: NONE	YIELD: 4 SERVINGS

INGREDIENTS

¼ cup lemon juice

¾ cup olive oil

2 tablespoons Dijon mustard

Salt and pepper to taste

4 cups chopped kale

4 ounces smoked salmon, sliced

1 cup fresh blueberries

⅓ cup shelled pistachios

2 large avocados, sliced

DIRECTIONS

1 To make dressing, place the lemon juice, olive oil, mustard, and salt and pepper in a blender or food processor and puree until smooth and creamy.

2 Place the kale in a large bowl and toss well with half of the dressing.

3 Add the remaining ingredients to the bowl and toss everything together.

4 Divide among four bowls. Serve with the remaining dressing and enjoy.

PER SERVING: *Calories 695; Fat 64g; Cholesterol 7mg; Sodium 364mg; Carbohydrate 25g (Dietary Fiber 12g, Sugar Alcohol 0g); Net Carbohydrate 13g; Protein 14g.*

Grilled Chicken Salad

PREP TIME: 10 MIN	COOK TIME: 10 MIN	YIELD: 2 SERVINGS

INGREDIENTS

1 tablespoon olive oil

1 teaspoon minced garlic

Salt and pepper to taste

2 medium boneless, skinless chicken breasts, pounded flat

1 cup chopped romaine lettuce

1 cup baby spinach, lightly packed

1 cup cherry tomatoes, quartered

1 cup red radicchio, chopped

¼ cup lemon turmeric vinaigrette (or your favorite keto lemon salad dressing)

1 avocado, halved, peeled, and pitted

DIRECTIONS

1 Preheat a grill pan over the stovetop or an outdoor grill to medium-high heat.

2 Mix the olive oil and minced garlic in a small bowl with salt and pepper.

3 Spread the oil mixture over the chicken breasts and then place them on the grill. Grill the chicken for 5 minutes; then flip and grill for another 5 minutes. Let the chicken breast sit for about 5 minutes before slicing.

4 While the chicken is resting, make the salad: Place the lettuce, spinach, tomatoes, and radicchio in a large bowl. Toss with the lemon turmeric vinaigrette and then divide between two bowls.

5 Top each salad with half an avocado and sliced grilled chicken breast. Enjoy!

PER SERVING: *Calories 539; Fat 34g; Cholesterol 64mg; Sodium 129mg; Carbohydrate 17g (Dietary Fiber 9g, Sugar Alcohol 0g); Net Carbohydrate 8g; Protein 43g.*

Tuna Salad Cucumber Boat

PREP TIME: 20 MIN | COOK TIME: NONE | YIELD: 4 SERVINGS

INGREDIENTS

2 medium cucumbers

2 (5-ounce) cans flaked tuna in water, drained

2 celery stalks, diced

½ cup chopped red bell pepper

½ cup plain Greek yogurt

½ teaspoon salt

½ teaspoon garlic powder

¼ teaspoon ground black pepper

1 teaspoon fresh chopped parsley

DIRECTIONS

1 Peel the cucumbers and slice them in half lengthwise. Use a spoon to scoop the seeds out of the center of the cucumber slices, hollowing out the cucumber into four boat-like shapes. Discard the seeds.

2 In a large bowl, combine the remaining ingredients. Mix well with a fork, mashing the tuna into flakes as you mix.

3 Scoop the tuna mixture into the hollowed-out cucumbers.

4 Serve chilled.

PER SERVING: *Calories 189; Fat 4g; Cholesterol 106mg; Sodium 425mg; Carbohydrate 5g (Dietary Fiber 1g, Sugar Alcohol 0g); Net Carbohydrate 4g; Protein 34g.*

Chicken Salad Lettuce Wraps

PREP TIME: 15 MIN | COOK TIME: NONE | YIELD: 4 SERVINGS

INGREDIENTS

½ cup plain Greek yogurt

1 celery stalk, chopped

¼ cup chopped green onion

1 tablespoon Dijon mustard

2 tablespoons lemon juice

Salt and pepper to taste

3 cups shredded rotisserie chicken

1 tomato, diced

1 large avocado, peeled, pitted, and chopped

12 butter lettuce leaves

DIRECTIONS

1 In a large bowl, combine the yogurt, celery, onion, mustard, lemon juice, and salt and pepper. Stir together well.

2 Add the shredded chicken to the bowl and mix well.

3 Add the tomato and avocado and stir gently so as not to mash the avocado.

4 Place the lettuce leaves on a clean work surface and scoop about ¼ cup of chicken salad into each leaf.

5 Serve while cold, three lettuce leaves per serving.

PER SERVING: *Calories 419; Fat 25g; Cholesterol 113mg; Sodium 180mg; Carbohydrate 8g (Dietary Fiber 4g, Sugar Alcohol 0g); Net Carbohydrate 4g; Protein 40g.*

Everything Crackers with Tuna Salad

PREP TIME: 15 MIN	COOK TIME: 30 MIN	YIELD: 6 SERVINGS

INGREDIENTS

½ cup ground flaxseeds

¾ cup almond flour

¼ teaspoon salt

2 tablespoons everything bagel seasoning

1 (5-ounce) can flaked tuna in water, drained

¼ cup mayonnaise

1 tablespoon Dijon mustard

¼ teaspoon garlic powder

Salt and pepper to taste

DIRECTIONS

1 Preheat the oven to 325 degrees and line a baking sheet with parchment paper.

2 In a large bowl, mix the flaxseeds, almond flour, salt, ½ cup of water, and everything bagel seasoning.

3 Let the mixture sit for about 10 minutes to thicken enough to form a ball.

4 Place the dough on the lined baking sheet and place a second piece of parchment paper on top of the dough.

5 Roll the dough between the two pieces of parchment until about ⅛-inch thick — the thinner, the better!

6 Score the dough several times to create your preferred cracker shapes (squares or rectangles) by pressing the knife three-fourths of the way down.

7 Bake for 30 minutes; the edges should turn brown.

8 Remove from the oven and let the crackers cool. Once cool, break the sheet into crackers by hand.

9 While the crackers are baking and cooling, make the tuna salad: Place the tuna, mayonnaise, Dijon mustard, and garlic powder in a bowl and mash together with a fork. Add salt and pepper to taste.

10 Serve the tuna dip with the crackers and enjoy!

PER SERVING: *Calories 245; Fat 19g; Cholesterol 34mg; Sodium 455mg; Carbohydrate 6g (Dietary Fiber 4g, Sugar Alcohol 0g); Net Carbohydrate 1g; Protein 15g.*

Chapter **13**

Lunches

Preparing a keto-friendly lunch can take a little planning. You can no longer run to the pizza store and grab a slice or pop into a deli to get a big, carb-loaded sandwich. Keto lunches are not necessarily difficult to make.

You will find the effort you put into your lunchtime routine extremely rewarding. Not only will you be eating nutritionally beneficial foods (let's face it, that slice of pizza you used to eat was not healthy), but you will also be creating meals that taste good. When you have an exciting keto lunch planned, your morning will fly by with anticipation for the next great meal.

We know that lunchtime is often rushed, but that doesn't mean you don't have time to make something delicious. You can rest assured that every recipe is high in fat, has a moderate amount of protein, and is low carb. Now, all you need to do is try out a few lunch recipes and discover which one is your favorite.

Avocado Salmon Chaffle Sandwich

PREP TIME: 10 MIN | COOK TIME: 24 MIN | YIELD: 2 SERVINGS

INGREDIENTS

2 tablespoons cream cheese

1 ounce goat cheese

½ teaspoon fresh dill

2 large eggs

1 cup shredded cheddar cheese

2 tablespoons almond flour

1 large avocado, peeled, pitted, and sliced

3 ounces smoked salmon

DIRECTIONS

1 In a bowl, combine the cream cheese, goat cheese, and dill.

2 Whisk the eggs, shredded cheddar, and almond flour in a separate large bowl.

3 Preheat a small waffle maker per the manufacturer's instructions.

4 Cook the cheese batter in the waffle maker. The batter should make four small waffles. Cook until the waffles are browned, about 5 to 6 minutes.

5 Spread equal amounts of the cream cheese mixture over two of the waffles.

6 Top each waffle with avocado slices and half of the smoked salmon.

7 Place the remaining two waffles on top of the salmon and enjoy!

PER SERVING: *Calories 630; Fat 51g; Cholesterol 125mg; Sodium 418mg; Carbohydrate 12g (Dietary Fiber 7g, Sugar Alcohol 0g); Net Carbohydrate 4g; Protein 34g.*

Spinach Feta Stuffed Chicken Skewers

PREP TIME: 15 MIN   COOK TIME: 20 MIN   YIELD: 4 SERVINGS

INGREDIENTS

1 tablespoon olive oil

1 clove garlic, minced

4 cups baby spinach, lightly packed

¼ cup fresh chopped basil

⅔ cup feta cheese crumbles

Salt and pepper

1½ pounds boneless, skinless chicken breast (about 4 breasts)

1 red bell pepper

1 yellow bell pepper

DIRECTIONS

1 Place the olive oil and garlic in a large skillet. Heat over medium heat and let the garlic cook for about 1 minute.

2 Add the spinach and basil to the pan with the garlic. Cover the pan and let the greens steam for 1 minute.

3 Remove the pan from the heat, stir in the feta cheese, and season with a little salt and pepper. Set aside.

4 Slice each chicken breast in half lengthwise. You should be able to cut each breast into about three fillets.

5 Use a meat mallet to gently pound the chicken fillets to that they are about ¼-inch thick.

6 Lay the fillets out on a clean work surface. Sprinkle with a little salt and pepper.

7 Scoop about half a tablespoon of spinach feta mixture onto the center of each chicken fillet. Spread the mixture across the fillet and then roll the chicken lengthwise into a spiral, enclosing the spinach filling. Repeat with all the chicken and filling.

8 Cut the bell peppers into eight pieces, removing the seeds.

9 Skewer the chicken rolls onto long metal skewers and skewer the red and yellow bell peppers onto separate skewers.

10 Preheat a grill to high heat.

11 Grill the chicken and pepper skewers for 8 minutes; flip and grill for another 8 minutes. Enjoy while hot!

PER SERVING: *Calories 330; Fat 13g; Cholesterol 146mg; Sodium 318mg; Carbohydrate 7g (Dietary Fiber 2g, Sugar Alcohol 0g); Net Carbohydrate 6g; Protein 43g.*

Grilled Lemon Chicken with Avocado Salad

PREP TIME: 45 MIN	COOK TIME: 14 MIN	YIELD: 4 SERVINGS

INGREDIENTS

¼ cup plus 2 tablespoons lemon juice, divided

¼ cup plus 2 tablespoons olive oil, divided

1 tablespoon lemon zest

Salt and pepper

4 (6-ounce) boneless, skinless chicken breasts

4 cups chopped romaine lettuce

2 cups cherry tomatoes, halved

2 large avocados, peeled, pitted, and sliced

DIRECTIONS

1 Place the lemon juice, olive oil, lemon zest, and a sprinkle of salt and pepper to the bowl. Set aside four tablespoons of the marinade and toss the chicken in the rest of the marinade. Let sit for at least 30 minutes.

2 Preheat a grill pan over the stovetop or an outdoor grill to medium–high.

3 Place the chicken breasts on the grill. Cook for 7 minutes; flip and cook for another 7 minutes. Discard any extra marinade.

4 Make the avocado salad while the chicken is cooking: Place the romaine in a large bowl along with the marinade set aside earlier. Add the tomatoes and avocado slices and toss everything together. Add a little salt and pepper and toss.

5 Divide the salad between four plates and add one grilled chicken breast per plate. Enjoy while the chicken is hot.

PER SERVING: *Calories 676; Fat 42g; Cholesterol 186mg; Sodium 133mg; Carbohydrate 15g (Dietary Fiber 9g, Sugar Alcohol 0g); Net Carbohydrate 6g; Protein 61g.*

Broccoli Chicken Crust Pizza with Avocado and Feta

PREP TIME: 10 MIN	COOK TIME: 30 MIN	YIELD: 4 SERVINGS

INGREDIENTS

10 ounces canned chicken

1 cup riced broccoli

1 large egg

½ cup grated Parmesan cheese

Salt and pepper

¾ cup feta cheese crumbles

1 cup sliced Baby Bella mushrooms

1 large avocado, pitted, peeled, and sliced

2 tablespoons chopped parsley

DIRECTIONS

1 Preheat the oven to 350 degrees and line a baking sheet with a silicone mat.

2 Drain the canned chicken, squeezing out as much juice as possible.

3 Spread the chicken on the prepared baking sheet and add the riced broccoli.

4 Bake the chicken and broccoli for 10 minutes to dry out the veggie and meat.

5 Remove the baking sheet from the oven and let cool for about 5 minutes.

6 Increase the oven temp to 475 degrees.

7 Place the chicken and broccoli to a large bowl and add the egg, Parmesan, and a little salt and pepper. Mix well to form a thick dough.

8 Place the chicken mixture back on the baking sheet and shape it into a round, ¼-inch-thick pizza crust.

9 Bake the crust for 10 minutes.

10 Remove the pan from the oven and spread the feta and mushrooms across the pizza. Return to the oven for another 10 minutes.

11 Remove the pizza from the oven and top it with the sliced avocado and parsley. Slice and serve!

PER SERVING: *Calories 343; Fat 23g; Cholesterol 119mg; Sodium 788mg; Carbohydrate 9g (Dietary Fiber 5g, Sugar Alcohol 0g); Net Carbohydrate 4g; Protein 27g.*

Almond Butter Shake

PREP TIME: 5 MIN	COOK TIME: NONE	YIELD: 1 SERVING

INGREDIENTS

1½ cups unsweetened almond milk

2 tablespoons almond butter

2 tablespoons ground flaxseeds

½ teaspoon ground cinnamon

1 tablespoon powdered erythritol

⅛ teaspoon almond extract

Pinch of salt

1 cup ice

DIRECTIONS

1 Place all the ingredients into a blender and puree until smooth.

2 Pour into a tall glass and enjoy.

PER SERVING: *Calories 329; Fat 28g; Cholesterol 0mg; Sodium 262mg; Carbohydrate 25g (Dietary Fiber 12g, Sugar Alcohol 12g); Net Carbohydrate 3g; Protein 11g.*

Keto Bacon Cheddar Egg Sandwich

PREP TIME: 5 MIN	COOK TIME: 10 MIN	YIELD: 2 SERVINGS

INGREDIENTS

6 large eggs

6 slices cooked bacon

6 slices cheddar cheese

Salt and pepper to taste

DIRECTIONS

1 Place the eggs in a large pot and add cold water so it covers the eggs by about an inch. Bring the water to a boil over medium heat; then turn off the heat, remove the pot from the stove, and let the eggs sit in the water for 10 minutes. Drain the water and run cold water over the eggs to stop them from cooking. Once cooled, peel the eggs.

2 Slice the cooked eggs in half lengthwise. The yolk may be slightly soft, but that is okay!

3 Place a strip of bacon and a piece of cheese on top of six of the egg halves and then top each "sandwich" with the other half of the egg, securing them together with a toothpick.

4 Sprinkle with salt and pepper and serve.

PER SERVING: *Calories 663; Fat 54g; Cholesterol 587mg; Sodium 943mg; Carbohydrate 2g (Dietary Fiber 0g, Sugar Alcohol 0g); Net Carbohydrate 2g; Protein 41g.*

Bacon-Wrapped Brussels Sprouts

PREP TIME: 15 MIN	COOK TIME: 30 MIN	YIELD: 2 SERVINGS

INGREDIENTS

20 whole Brussels sprouts

10 strips of bacon, uncooked

DIRECTIONS

1 Preheat the oven to 375 degrees and line a rimmed baking sheet with aluminum foil.

2 Cut each strip of bacon in half lengthwise.

3 Wrap each Brussels sprout with a half strip of bacon, placing the wrapped sprout on the prepared baking sheet.

4 Bake for 30 minutes so the bacon is crispy and the sprout is soft.

5 Enjoy while hot.

PER SERVING: *Calories 331; Fat 25g; Cholesterol 36mg; Sodium 412mg; Carbohydrate 18g (Dietary Fiber 7g, Sugar Alcohol 0g); Net Carbohydrate 10g; Protein 13g.*

Cauliflower Hash Browns

PREP TIME: 10 MIN	COOK TIME: 27 MIN	YIELD: 2 SERVINGS

INGREDIENTS

3 cups riced cauliflower

1 large egg

1 cup shredded cheddar cheese

¼ cup chopped fresh green onions

Salt and pepper

¼ teaspoon garlic powder

DIRECTIONS

1 Preheat the oven to 400 degrees and line a baking sheet with aluminum foil. Spray the foil sheet well with cooking spray.

2 Microwave the cauliflower rice for 2 minutes, uncovered.

3 Let the cauliflower rice cool, and then use a piece of cheese-cloth to squeeze the moisture out of the cauliflower. This will make the hash browns crispier.

4 Place the dried cauliflower rice into a large bowl.

5 Whisk the egg and pour it over the cauliflower.

6 Add the cheese, green onions, a little salt and pepper, and garlic powder and stir well.

7 Scoop the dough into eight balls. Roll and press each one flat to be about 1/4-inch thick. Place the patties on the prepared baking sheet, spacing them at least an inch apart.

8 Bake the hash browns for 20 minutes.

9 Remove the baking sheet and turn the oven up to broil. Flip the hash browns and place the baking sheet under the broiler for 5 minutes to brown the tops.

10 Enjoy while hot.

PER SERVING: *Calories 171; Fat 13g; Cholesterol 138mg; Sodium 641mg; Carbohydrate 5g (Dietary Fiber 2g, Sugar Alcohol 0g); Net Carbohydrate 3g; Protein 10g.*

Garlic Chicken Fritters

PREP TIME: 10 MIN	COOK TIME: 10 MIN	YIELD: 4 SERVINGS

INGREDIENTS

1½ pounds boneless, skinless chicken breast

2 large eggs

⅓ cup mayonnaise

½ cup almond flour

½ teaspoon xanthan gum

1 cup shredded mozzarella cheese

1 tablespoon minced garlic

Salt and pepper

2 tablespoons olive oil

DIRECTIONS

1 Chop the chicken breast into small pieces; ¼-inch cubes work best (the smaller, the better!). Place the chicken into a large bowl.

2 Add the eggs, mayo, almond flour, xanthan gum, mozzarella, garlic, and a sprinkle of salt and pepper to the bowl and toss with the chicken. Cover and let sit in the fridge for 2 hours. This will give the fritter batter time to thicken.

3 Place the olive oil in a large skillet and heat over medium-high heat. Scoop the chicken fritter batter into the hot oil, making tablespoon-sized scoops. Fry the fritters for 3 minutes; then flip and fry for another 3 minutes. The fritters should be golden brown.

4 Remove the fritters from the skillet and place them on a paper towel to drain. Cook the remaining chicken fritters. Enjoy while warm!

PER SERVING: *Calories 666; Fat 51g; Cholesterol 210mg; Sodium 402mg; Carbohydrate 6g (Dietary Fiber 2g, Sugar Alcohol 0g); Net Carbohydrate 4g; Protein 47g.*

Keto Corn Dogs with Avocado

| PREP TIME: 20 MIN | COOK TIME: 16 MIN | YIELD: 6 SERVINGS |

INGREDIENTS

6 beef hot dogs

3½ cups shredded mozzarella cheese

1½ cups almond flour

1 large egg

¼ teaspoon garlic powder

Salt and pepper

1 teaspoon xanthan gum

1 teaspoon baking powder

2 large avocados, for serving

DIRECTIONS

1 Preheat the oven to 400 degrees and line a baking sheet with aluminum foil. Spray the foil sheet well with cooking spray.

2 Stick a wooden skewer into each hot dog and then place the hot dogs on a plate to set aside.

3 Put the shredded mozzarella into a bowl and microwave for about 30 seconds. Stir and microwave for another 30 seconds. Repeat this step until the cheese is completely melted.

4 Add the almond flour and egg to the smooth, melted cheese, stirring quickly so as not to cook the egg.

5 Add the garlic powder, a little salt and pepper, xanthan gum, and baking powder to the bowl and stir well.

6 Place the thick cheese dough on a piece of parchment paper and then place a second piece of parchment paper on top of the dough. Roll the dough between the parchment paper until it is about ¼-inch thick.

7 Slice the dough into six strips and then wrap each piece of dough around a hot dog. Try to seal the dough at the seam so the hot dog is completely enclosed in the dough.

8 Place the corn dogs on the prepared baking sheet and bake for 15 minutes, turning halfway through so they are evenly golden brown.

9 Serve while hot with fresh sliced avocado sprinkled with a little salt and pepper.

PER SERVING: *Calories 587; Fat 48g; Cholesterol 93mg; Sodium 994mg; Carbohydrate 18g (Dietary Fiber 8g, Sugar Alcohol 0g); Net Carbohydrate 10g; Protein 26g.*

Cauliflower Mac and Cheese

PREP TIME: 15 MIN | **COOK TIME: 40 MIN** | **YIELD: 6 SERVINGS**

INGREDIENTS

8 cups chopped cauliflower florets

2 tablespoons unsalted butter

¼ cup chopped white onion

1 teaspoon psyllium husk powder

2 cups whole milk

Salt and pepper

2 cups shredded cheddar cheese

DIRECTIONS

1 Preheat the oven to 400 degrees. Lightly grease a 9-x-13-inch baking dish.

2 Place the cauliflower in a large pot and add about 2 cups of water. Bring the water to a boil and cover the pot.

3 Steam the cauliflower for 5 minutes. Drain the water and set the cauliflower aside in a large bowl.

4 Place the butter in a large pot and melt over medium heat.

5 Add the onion to the pot and sauté for about 3 minutes.

6 Add the psyllium husk powder to the pot and whisk.

7 Pour the milk into the pot, whisking constantly.

8 Bring the milk to a boil and lower the heat to a simmer. Simmer the milk for about 2 minutes to thicken.

9 Remove the milk from the heat. Add a sprinkle of salt and pepper and the cheese. Whisk until the cheese melts into the mixture and is nice and smooth.

10 Add the steamed cauliflower back into the pot and stir the cauliflower into the cheese sauce.

11 Pour the cauliflower into the baking dish and place the pan into the oven. Bake for about 25 minutes or until the sauce bubbles around the edges. Enjoy while hot.

PER SERVING: *Calories 279; Fat 20g; Cholesterol 57mg; Sodium 321mg; Carbohydrate 13g (Dietary Fiber 4g, Sugar Alcohol 0g); Net Carbohydrate 9g; Protein 14g.*

Pumpkin Chia Muffin

PREP TIME: 10 MIN	COOK TIME: 24 MIN	YIELD: 6 SERVINGS

INGREDIENTS

4 large eggs

½ cup pumpkin puree

4 tablespoons unsalted butter, melted

⅓ cup granular erythritol

1 tablespoon chia seeds

2 teaspoons vanilla extract

⅓ cup coconut flour

2 teaspoons pumpkin pie spice

1 teaspoon baking powder

DIRECTIONS

1 Preheat the oven to 350 degrees. Line a muffin pan with six paper muffin cups.

2 In a medium-sized bowl, whisk together the eggs, pumpkin puree, melted butter, granular erythritol, chia seeds, and vanilla extract.

3 Fold in the coconut flour, pumpkin pie spice, and baking powder.

4 Scoop the batter into the paper muffin cups, filling them about three-fourths of the way to the top.

5 Bake in the oven for 24 minutes. Let cool on a cooling rack, and then enjoy.

PER SERVING: *Calories 160; Fat 12g; Cholesterol 127mg; Sodium 117mg; Carbohydrate 18g (Dietary Fiber 4g, Sugar Alcohol 11g); Net Carbohydrate 4g; Protein 5g.*

Meat and Cheese–Stuffed Tomatoes

PREP TIME: 20 MIN	COOK TIME: 8 MIN	YIELD: 4 SERVINGS

INGREDIENTS

1 pound ground sausage, no casings

12 medium tomatoes

2 ounces Monterey Jack cheese, thinly sliced

1 cup shredded mozzarella cheese

3 tablespoons olive oil

1 tablespoon fresh chopped parsley

DIRECTIONS

1 Put the ground sausage in a skillet and cook over medium-high heat. Break up the sausage as it cooks with a spatula.

2 Once the sausage is golden brown, remove the pan from the heat. Set aside.

3 Preheat the oven to 400 degrees and line a baking sheet with aluminum foil.

4 Cut a tiny slice off the bottom of each tomato so the tomato can stand up straight. Slice off the top of each tomato and then use a small spoon to scoop out the seeds and most of the center, making a tomato bowl. Place the hollow tomatoes upright on the prepared baking sheet.

5 Arrange the thin slices of Monterey Jack cheese on the inside of the tomato, placing the slices around the edges of the tomato "bowl."

6 Fill each tomato with the cooked sausage.

7 Top each tomato with shredded mozzarella cheese.

8 Use a pastry brush to brush the olive oil on the outside of each tomato.

9 Bake the tomatoes in the oven for about 8 minutes or until the cheese has melted and begins to turn golden brown.

10 Remove the tomatoes from the oven and garnish with fresh parsley. Enjoy while hot.

PER SERVING: *Calories 676; Fat 56g; Cholesterol 77mg; Sodium 1,093mg; Carbohydrate 17g (Dietary Fiber 4g, Sugar Alcohol 0g); Net Carbohydrate 13g; Protein 29g.*

Bacon, Brussels Sprouts, and Egg Skillet

PREP TIME: 10 MIN	COOK TIME: 21 MIN	YIELD: 4 SERVINGS

INGREDIENTS

½ pound thick-cut bacon

¼ cup chopped shallots

½ pound halved Brussels sprouts

1 medium zucchini, sliced

Salt and pepper

¼ cup Gruyère cheese

¼ cup crumbled Parmesan cheese

8 large eggs

DIRECTIONS

1 Place the oven rack about 6 inches away from the heating element and preheat the broiler.

2 Cook the bacon in a large, oven-safe, cast-iron skillet. Cook for about 5 minutes; flip and cook for another 5 minutes. Remove the bacon from the pan and chop it into smaller pieces. Return the bacon grease pan to the stovetop.

3 Add the shallots to the pan and sauté for 1 minute.

4 Add the Brussels sprouts and zucchini slices to the pan and toss in the bacon grease. Cook for 5 minutes, tossing occasionally.

5 Sprinkle the veggies with salt and pepper and then stir in both cheeses. Remove the pan from the heat.

6 Crack the eggs into the pan, keeping the yolks whole if possible. Try to crack the eggs in different spots in the skillet so that the yolks are evenly distributed around the skillet.

7 Place the skillet under the broiler and cook for about 4 to 5 minutes until the egg whites are set.

8 Slice and enjoy while hot.

PER SERVING: *Calories 500; Fat 37g; Cholesterol 381mg; Sodium 1,453mg; Carbohydrate 9g (Dietary Fiber 3g, Sugar Alcohol 0g); Net Carbohydrate 6g; Protein 37g.*

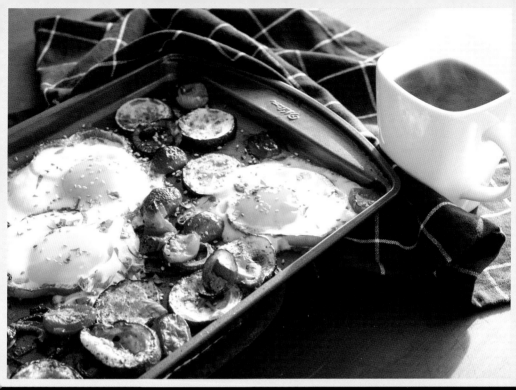

Sheet Pan Breakfast Bake (Chapter 9)

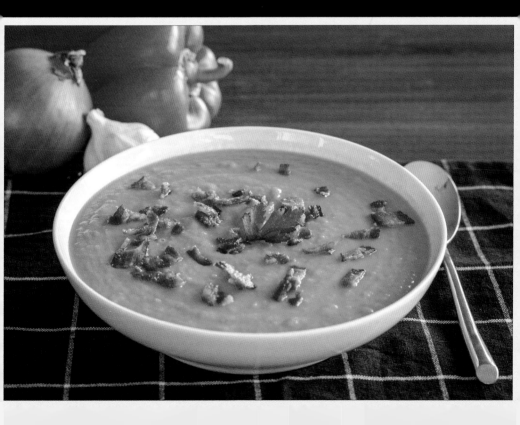

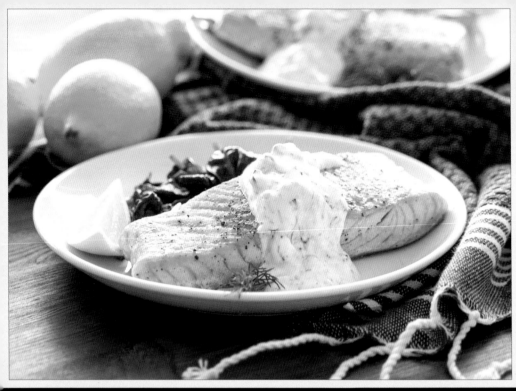

Seared Salmon with Cream Remoulade Sauce (Chapter 14)

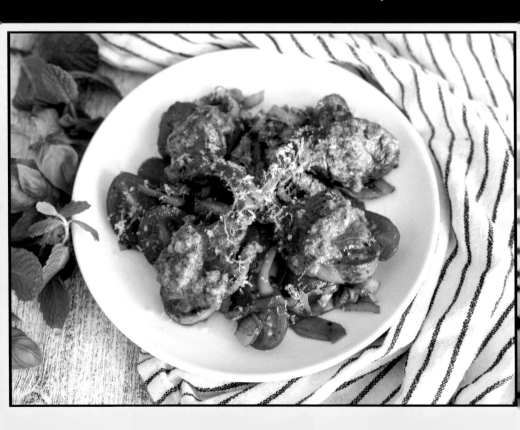

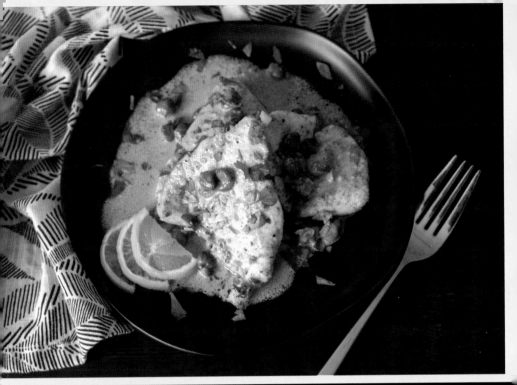

Creamy Chicken Picatta (Chapter 15)

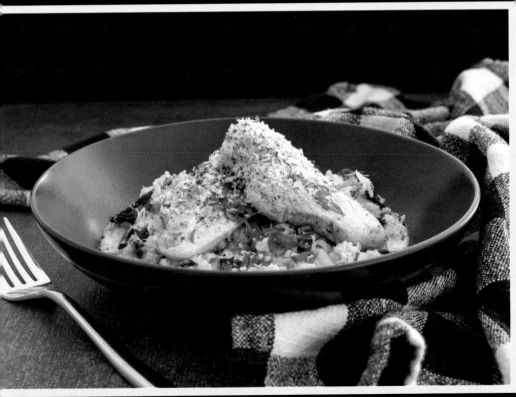

Baked Chicken with Creamy Cauliflower Rice (Chapter 15)

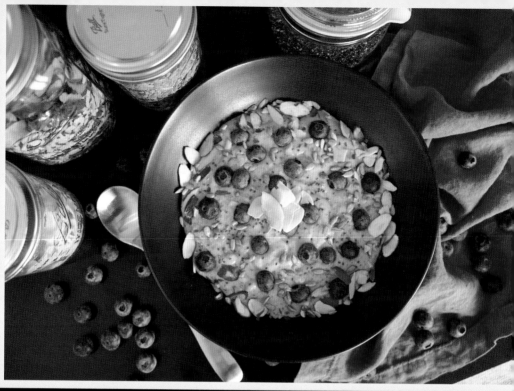

Super Green Smoothie Bowl (Chapter 18)

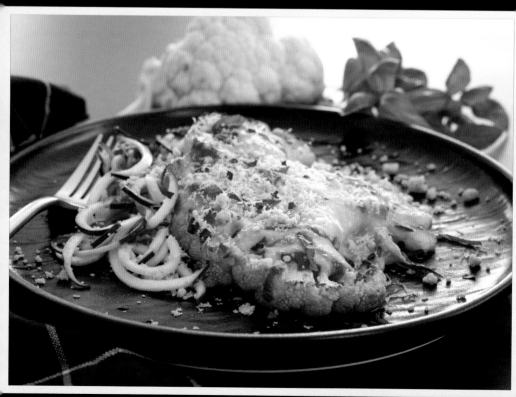

Cauliflower Parmesan and Zoodles with Tomato Sauce (Chapter 18)

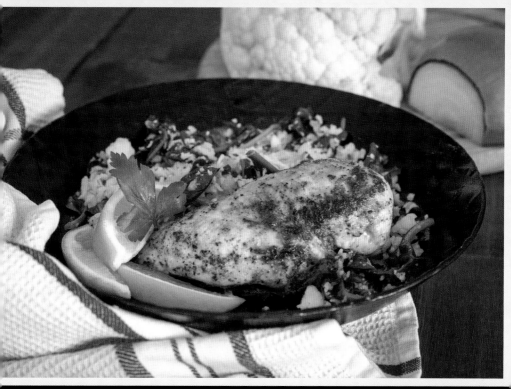

Air Fryer Chicken with Cauliflower Rice (Chapter 20)

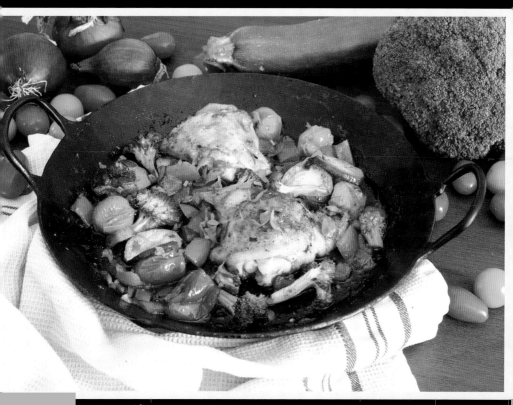

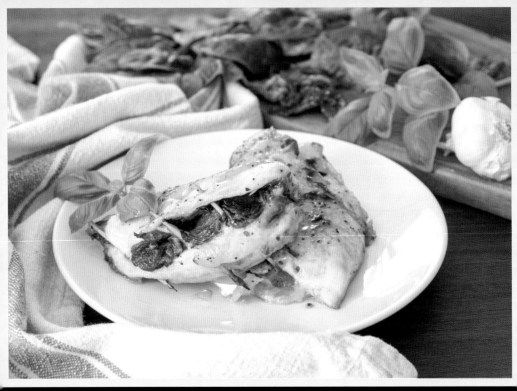

Caprese Stuffed Chicken (Chapter 20)

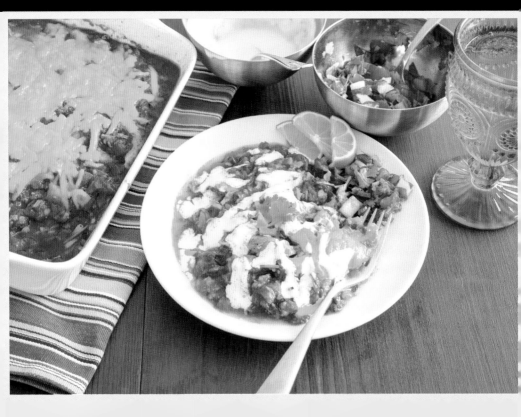

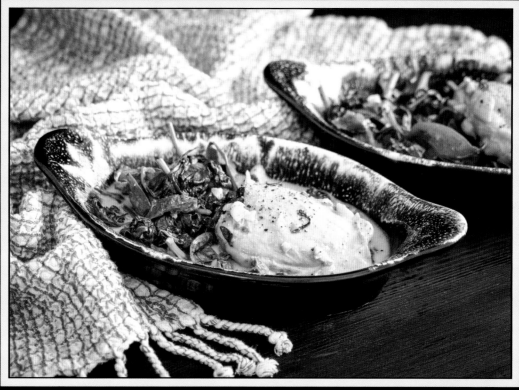

Creamy Parmesan Chicken with Spinach (Chapter 22)

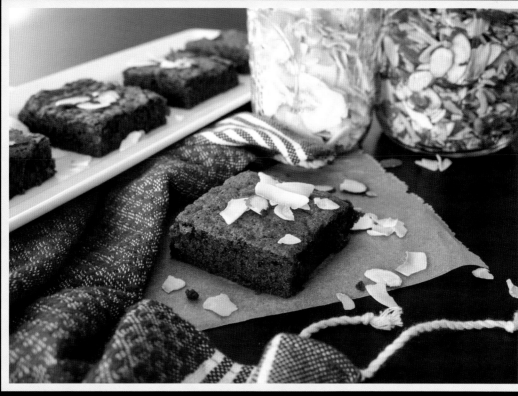

Dark Chocolate Brownies (Chapter 25)

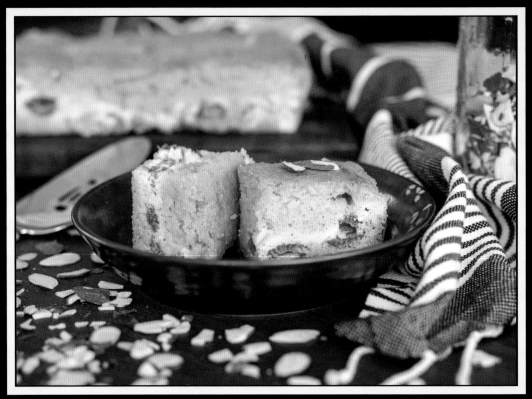

Raspberry Almond Cake (Chapter 25)

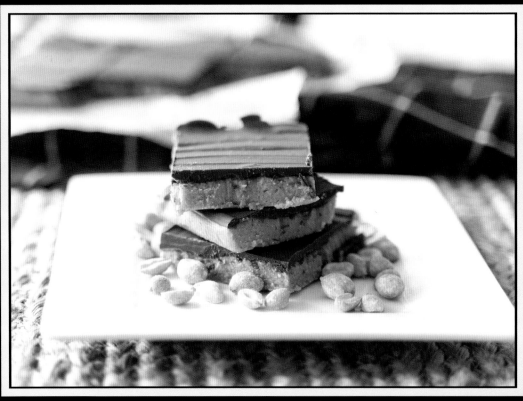

No-Bake Peanut Butter Bars (Chapter 25)

Chapter **14**

Fish Dinners

You don't usually have to worry about carbs when eating fish. Fish, on its own, does not contain carbs but is made up of healthy fats and lean proteins. The trick is to turn that plain fish filet into a dinner you will adore.

While lots of fish are high in omega-3 fatty acids, fish is often lower in fat. Fish is not as high in fat as pork or beef, for example, so a keto dieter will need to find a way to boost the fat content of the fish. Luckily, there are plenty of ways to do this!

Sautéing fish in ghee, oil, or butter is an effortless way to increase the meal's fat content. You can also choose naturally oily fish such as wild-caught salmon or mackerel. Keeping the skin on the fish helps you stick to the keto macros because of how fatty the skin is. We love playing around with sauces and glazes, pouring the rich buttery sauce over freshly fried fish. You can't go wrong with a creamy keto sauce!

If you are a fish lover, you will appreciate these tasty keto fish dinners. They help turn lean fish into a high-fat keto meal. We created recipes using a wide variety of fishes. You have plenty of options for keto seafood, from Mahi Mahi to shrimp.

Creamy Lemon Mahi Mahi

| PREP TIME: 10 MIN | COOK TIME: 15 MIN | YIELD: 4 SERVINGS |

INGREDIENTS

4 (6-ounce) Mahi Mahi filets

Salt

¼ teaspoon lemon pepper seasoning

2 medium lemons

4 tablespoons unsalted butter

2 tablespoons minced garlic

½ cup heavy cream

2 tablespoons fresh chopped parsley

2 cups baby spinach, lightly packed

DIRECTIONS

1 Sprinkle the Mahi Mahi with a sprinkle of salt and the lemon pepper seasoning.

2 Thinly slice one of the lemons and set aside.

3 Juice the second lemon and remove any seeds.

4 Place the butter in a large skillet and melt over medium-high heat.

5 Add the Mahi Mahi filets to the hot butter in the pan and sear each side for 4 minutes. The fish should have a golden-brown crust and no longer be opaque.

6 Remove the fish from the pan and set it aside on a plate.

7 Add the lemon juice and lemon slices to the same skillet with the leftover melted butter.

8 Add the garlic and stir. Cook the sauce for about a minute.

9 Add the heavy cream and bring the sauce to a simmer. Simmer for about 2 minutes to thicken the sauce.

10 Add the parsley and return the fish filets back into the pan. Cook for 1 minute to reheat.

11 Serve the fish over a bed of spinach with the sauce spooned over each filet.

PER SERVING: *Calories 359; Fat 24g; Cholesterol 192mg; Sodium 259mg; Carbohydrate 6g (Dietary Fiber 1g, Sugar Alcohol 0g); Net Carbohydrate 4g; Protein 34g.*

Cauliflower Shrimp Fried Rice

PREP TIME: 10 MIN	COOK TIME: 17 MIN	YIELD: 4 SERVINGS

INGREDIENTS

5 cups cauliflower florets

2 tablespoons sesame oil, divided

1 pound shrimp, peeled and deveined

Salt and pepper

2 large eggs, whisked

¼ cup chopped green onions

1 tablespoon minced garlic

½ cup diced red bell pepper

2 tablespoons soy sauce

DIRECTIONS

1 Place the cauliflower florets in a food processor and pulse until it resembles rice. Set aside.

2 Heat 1 tablespoon of the sesame oil in a large skillet or wok over medium-high heat.

3 Add the shrimp to the pan and season with salt and pepper.

4 Cook the shrimp for 3 minutes; flip and cook for another 2 minutes.

5 Remove the shrimp from the pan and set aside.

6 Pour the eggs into the pan that the shrimp cooked in. Scramble quickly with a spatula, cooking for about 1 minute. Remove from the pan and set aside as well.

7 Return the skillet to the heat and add the remaining 1 tablespoon of sesame oil.

8 Add the cauliflower rice to the skillet and cook for about 5 minutes, stirring every so often.

9 Make some space in the skillet and add the green onions to the skillet along with the garlic and bell pepper. Sauté for about 2 to 3 minutes until fragrant.

10 Add the scrambled eggs, shrimp, and soy sauce to the skillet and toss everything together well.

11 Divide among four bowls and enjoy hot.

PER SERVING: *Calories 219; Fat 10g; Cholesterol 223mg; Sodium 1,154mg; Carbohydrate 10g (Dietary Fiber 3g, Sugar Alcohol 0g); Net Carbohydrate 7g; Protein 22g.*

Smoked Paprika Salmon with Grilled Veggies

PREP TIME: 10 MIN	COOK TIME: 15 MIN	YIELD: 4 SERVINGS

INGREDIENTS

4 (8-ounce) salmon filets, skin on

3 tablespoons olive oil, divided

1 teaspoon salt plus more for veggies

1 tablespoon smoked paprika

1 pound asparagus spears

2 long red peppers, seeds removed, halved lengthwise

1 medium zucchini, sliced

Pepper, for veggies

DIRECTIONS

1 Preheat a grill or pan to medium-high heat.

2 Pat the salmon filets dry. Coat both sides of the salmon in 2 tablespoons of olive oil and then sprinkle the salt and paprika over the salmon. Rub the seasonings into the fish.

3 Place the seasoned salmon filets on the hot grill and cook for about 8 minutes. Flip and cook for another 4 minutes.

4 Remove the salmon from the grill and place on four plates.

5 Toss the asparagus spears, red pepper slices, and zucchini slices in a large bowl with the remaining 1 tablespoon of olive oil. Season the veggies with a little salt and pepper.

6 Spread the seasoned veggies across the grill grates or on a veggie basket and grill for 2 minutes. Flip and grill for 1 more minute.

7 Serve the salmon and grilled veggies while hot.

PER SERVING: *Calories 615; Fat 50g; Cholesterol 129mg; Sodium 187mg; Carbohydrate 10g (Dietary Fiber 5g, Sugar Alcohol 0g); Net Carbohydrate 6g; Protein 50g.*

Herbed Halibut with Lemon Garlic Spinach

PREP TIME: 5 MIN | COOK TIME: 15 MIN | YIELD: 4 SERVINGS

INGREDIENTS

½ teaspoon dried rosemary

1 teaspoon Italian seasoning

¼ teaspoon crushed red pepper flakes

4 (6-ounce) halibut filets

1 tablespoon unsalted butter

1 tablespoon olive oil

1 tablespoon minced garlic

8 cups baby spinach, lightly packed

2 tablespoons lemon juice

DIRECTIONS

1 In a small bowl, stir together the rosemary, Italian seasoning, and crushed red pepper flakes.

2 Coat the halibut filets in the seasoning mix.

3 Put the butter in a large skillet and heat over medium-high heat. Add the halibut to the skillet and sear for 5 minutes. Flip and cook for another 5 minutes.

4 Remove the halibut from the pan and set aside.

5 Add the olive oil to the same pan that you cooked the fish in.

6 Add the garlic to the pan and sauté for 1 minute.

7 Add the spinach to the sauté pan and cook for 2 minutes, occasionally stirring to wilt the spinach.

8 Add the lemon juice to the pan with the spinach and toss.

9 Divide the spinach among four plates and place a seared halibut filet on top. Enjoy hot.

PER SERVING: *Calories 230; Fat 9g; Cholesterol 91mg; Sodium 164mg; Carbohydrate 4g (Dietary Fiber 2g, Sugar Alcohol 0g); Net Carbohydrate 2g; Protein 9g.*

Pesto Zoodles with Garlic Butter Shrimp

PREP TIME: 10 MIN	COOK TIME: 10 MIN	YIELD: 4 SERVINGS

INGREDIENTS

2 medium zucchinis, ends trimmed

2 tablespoons unsalted butter

4 teaspoons minced garlic

24 shrimp, peeled and deveined

Salt and pepper

½ cup pesto sauce

2 tablespoons grated Parmesan cheese, divided

DIRECTIONS

1 Cut the zucchini using a spiralizer to make zucchini noodles.

2 Place the zoodles in a sieve and sprinkle with some salt. Set aside.

3 Place the butter in a large skillet and heat over medium heat.

4 Once the butter has melted, add the garlic to the pan and sauté for 1 minute.

5 Add the shrimp to the skillet and sprinkle with salt and pepper. Sauté the shrimp for 2 minutes; flip and cook for another 2 minutes. Remove the shrimp from the pan and set aside.

6 Add the zoodles to the pan and toss in the leftover butter. Cook in the skillet for 2 minutes.

7 Add the pesto to the skillet and toss the noodles in the pesto.

8 Divide the pesto zoodles among four bowls and top each with six garlic shrimp, a sprinkle of salt and pepper, and ½ tablespoon Parmesan. Serve hot.

PER SERVING: *Calories 360; Fat 30g; Cholesterol 86mg; Sodium 1,058mg; Carbohydrate 10g (Dietary Fiber 2g, Sugar Alcohol 0g); Net Carbohydrate 8g; Protein 14g.*

Seared Salmon with Cream Remoulade Sauce

PREP TIME: 10 MIN	COOK TIME: 10 MIN	YIELD: 2 SERVINGS

INGREDIENTS

1 cup plain Greek yogurt

2 tablespoons chopped capers

1 tablespoon fresh chopped dill

1 teaspoon lemon juice

Salt and pepper

1 pound salmon filets

2 tablespoons olive oil

6 cups baby spinach, lightly packed

¼ teaspoon garlic powder

DIRECTIONS

1   Make the yogurt remoulade sauce: In a small bowl, stir together the yogurt, capers, dill, lemon juice, and a sprinkle of salt and pepper. Set aside.

2   Sprinkle the salmon with salt and pepper on both sides.

3   Place the olive oil in a large skillet and heat over medium-high heat.

4   Add the salmon to the skillet and cook for 3 minutes. Flip and cook for another 3 minutes. Remove the salmon from the skillet and place on two serving plates.

5   Place the skillet back on the stovetop over medium-low heat.

6   Add the spinach to the skillet along with the garlic powder and season with salt and pepper. Toss to wilt (about 1 to 2 minutes of cooking time).

7   Divide the cooked spinach between the two plates.

8   Scoop the yogurt remoulade sauce over the salmon and spinach and enjoy while warm.

PER SERVING: *Calories 741; Fat 52g; Cholesterol 72mg; Sodium 238mg; Carbohydrate 9g (Dietary Fiber 2g, Sugar Alcohol 0g); Net Carbohydrate 7g; Protein 60g.*

Poached Salmon with Garlic Butter Spinach

PREP TIME: 5 MIN	COOK TIME: 10 MIN	YIELD: 2 SERVINGS

INGREDIENTS

½ cup vegetable broth

1 sprig parsley

¼ cup chopped onion

1 pound salmon filets, boneless

½ teaspoon salt

¼ teaspoon ground black pepper

4 tablespoons unsalted butter

4 cloves garlic, minced

½ pound baby spinach, lightly packed

2 lemon wedges

DIRECTIONS

1 Pour ½ cup of water in a skillet and add the vegetable broth, parsley, and onions. Bring to a simmer over medium heat.

2 Sprinkle the salmon filets with the salt and pepper.

3 Place the salmon in the pan of poaching liquid and cover it. Cook for 5 to 10 minutes, longer for thicker pieces of salmon.

4 While the salmon cooks, make the spinach. Place the butter in another large skillet and melt over medium heat.

5 Add the garlic and sauté for 2 minutes.

6 Add the baby spinach and stir, wilting the spinach in the garlic butter.

7 Divide the spinach between two plates and top with the poached salmon. Squeeze the lemon wedges over each plate and then enjoy.

PER SERVING: *Calories 721; Fat 54g; Cholesterol 93mg; Sodium 120mg; Carbohydrate 9g (Dietary Fiber 3g, Sugar Alcohol 0g); Net Carbohydrate 6g; Protein 51g.*

Smoked Salmon Poke Bowl

PREP TIME: 25 MIN	COOK TIME: 5 MIN	YIELD: 2 SERVINGS

INGREDIENTS

Salmon:

1 pound sushi grade salmon cut into 1-inch cubes

¼ cup coconut aminos

1 teaspoon rice wine vinegar

1 teaspoon Sriracha

1 teaspoon sesame oil

Pickled Cucumbers:

½ cup rice wine vinegar

⅓ cup low-carb pancake syrup

1 teaspoon salt

½ teaspoon red chili flakes

1 cucumber, sliced

Sauce:

2 tablespoons Sriracha

2 tablespoons plain Greek yogurt

Bowl:

1 cup shredded red cabbage

1 medium avocado, sliced

DIRECTIONS

1 Place the cubed salmon in a medium-sized bowl and add the coconut aminos, rice wine vinegar, Sriracha, and sesame oil. Toss everything together well. Cover the bowl and place the salmon in the fridge to marinate for 30 minutes.

2 Make the pickled cucumbers: Place the vinegar, pancake syrup, salt, and red chili flakes in a saucepan and bring to a boil over medium-high heat. Remove the pot from the heat and add the cucumber slices. Let the cucumbers sit for 10 minutes.

3 Make the sauce: In a separate small bowl, whisk together the Sriracha and Greek yogurt.

4 Divide the shredded cabbage and sliced avocado between two bowls. Add the marinated salmon and the pickled cucumbers to each bowl.

5 Drizzle the creamy sriracha sauce over each bowl, and then enjoy fresh!

PER SERVING: *Calories 774; Fat 49g; Cholesterol 63mg; Sodium 1,150mg; Carbohydrate 42g (Dietary Fiber 20g, Sugar Alcohol 7g); Net Carbohydrate 16g; Protein 51g.*

Chapter **15**

Meat Dinners

You may not always have time to prepare a deluxe breakfast or lunch, but there's a good chance you can put some effort into your dinner. Most of us have more time in the evening to make dinner, and you may also look forward to spending some time in the kitchen. It can be fun to cook and prepare healthy, flavorful foods that fill your belly and power your body.

When you first start your keto diet, almost everything you cook will be new. It can be tricky to re-learn how to cook using low-carb methods and ingredients. Some people get stuck in a keto dinner rut, repeatedly preparing the same foods because that's all they know how to make. We urge you to make at least one new keto recipe per week. Give some new things a try and test out your culinary skills! You'll be surprised by how much you can do in the kitchen and how many fantastic culinary creations you can make.

This chapter provides plenty of yummy, filling, meat-based keto dinners. You may come across new ingredients or ways to use some of your favorite classic ingredients. You'll be using a lot more butter in your cooking. Time to get out that frying pan and start preparing some incredible keto dinners.

Ricotta Sausage Skillet

PREP TIME: 10 MIN | COOK TIME: 15 MIN | YIELD: 4 SERVINGS

INGREDIENTS

3 tablespoons olive oil

1 tablespoon minced garlic

1 white onion, chopped

8 cooked chicken sausage links, cut into 1-inch slices

3 cups kale, finely chopped

2 teaspoons fresh chopped thyme

Salt and pepper

1 tablespoon lemon juice

1 cup fresh ricotta cheese

DIRECTIONS

1 Place the olive oil into a large cast-iron skillet and heat over medium heat.

2 Add the garlic and onions to the skillet and cook for 4 to 5 minutes, stirring occasionally.

3 Add the sausage slices to the skillet and cook for about 5 minutes.

4 Add the chopped kale, thyme, a sprinkle of salt and pepper, and lemon juice to the skillet. Stir and cook for 3 to 4 minutes to wilt the kale.

5 Scoop the ricotta into the skillet and stir to make a cheesy sauce or leave the ricotta on top as a tasty garnish.

6 Divide among four plates and enjoy.

PER SERVING: *Calories 414; Fat 29g; Cholesterol 130mg; Sodium 928mg; Carbohydrate 12g (Dietary Fiber 2g, Sugar Alcohol 0g); Net Carbohydrate 10g; Protein 29g.*

Baked Chicken with Creamy Cauliflower Rice

PREP TIME: 15 MIN	COOK TIME: 30 MIN	YIELD: 4 SERVINGS

INGREDIENTS

4 boneless, skinless chicken breasts (about 1½ pounds)

¼ cup melted unsalted butter, divided

1½ teaspoons salt, divided

1 teaspoon ground black pepper, divided

½ teaspoon garlic powder

½ cup chopped white onion

1 cauliflower head, grated or riced in a food processor

½ cup heavy cream

1 cup grated Parmesan cheese

2 cups baby spinach, lightly packed

DIRECTIONS

1   Preheat the oven to 450 degrees.

2   Place the chicken breasts in a large casserole dish or rimmed baking sheet.

3   Brush the chicken breasts evenly with 1 tablespoon of the melted butter.

4   Sprinkle the chicken breasts with 1 teaspoon salt, ½ teaspoon pepper, and garlic powder.

5   Bake the chicken in the oven for 18 to 20 minutes. The internal temperature of the chicken should be 165 degrees on a meat thermometer.

6   Remove the chicken from the oven, cover with aluminum foil and let rest in the dish for 10 minutes.

7   While the chicken is resting, make the cauliflower rice. Add the remaining butter to a large skillet along with the onions. Sauté for 5 minutes to soften the onions.

8   Add the cauliflower rice and stir.

9   Add the heavy cream and Parmesan cheese and stir well. Bring the mix to a simmer; then remove from the heat.

10   Stir in the spinach to wilt.

11   Scoop the rice onto four plates and serve with a roasted chicken breast. Enjoy while hot.

PER SERVING: *Calories 623; Fat 43g; Cholesterol 200mg; Sodium 393mg; Carbohydrate 10g (Dietary Fiber 3g, Sugar Alcohol 0g); Net Carbohydrate 7g; Protein 47g.*

Pesto Skillet Lamb and Veggies

PREP TIME: 10 MIN	COOK TIME: 22 MIN	YIELD: 4 SERVINGS

INGREDIENTS

5 tablespoons olive oil, divided

Salt and pepper

3 cloves garlic, minced and divided

¼ cup pine nuts

1 cup fresh basil

1½ cups fresh mint

½ cup Parmesan cheese

2 pounds lamb chops, cut individually (about 8 chops)

1 large leek, sliced thinly

2 cups cherry tomatoes, halved

DIRECTIONS

1　Add 1 tablespoon of olive oil to a large skillet on medium-high heat.

2　Season the lamb chops with a little salt and pepper on both sides.

3　Once the skillet is hot, add half of the lamb chops to the skillet. Sear them for 4 minutes on each side. Repeat with the remaining lamb chops. Set the lamb chops aside.

4　Make the pesto: Place two-thirds of the garlic, all the pine nuts, basil, mint, and Parmesan cheese in a food processor. Pulse the food processor to puree the pesto well, streaming in 4 tablespoons of olive oil. Once a smooth pesto forms, turn off the food processor and set the mint pesto aside.

5　To the same skillet, add the leeks. Sauté the leeks for about 5 minutes to soften.

6　Add the tomatoes and the remaining garlic to the skillet and cook for about a minute to soften.

7　Add the lamb chops back to the skillet with the veggies for about 1 minute.

8　Divide the lamb, tomatoes, and leeks among four plates and top with the mint pesto. Enjoy hot.

PER SERVING: *Calories 1,146; Fat 105g; Cholesterol 182mg; Sodium 335mg; Carbohydrate 10g (Dietary Fiber 3g, Sugar Alcohol 0g); Net Carbohydrate 8g; Protein 40g.*

Parmesan Pork Roast with Asparagus

PREP TIME: 15 MIN	COOK TIME: 45 MIN	YIELD: 6 SERVINGS

INGREDIENTS

1 tablespoon olive oil

1 teaspoon dried thyme

¾ cup Parmesan cheese

Salt and pepper

2 to 3 pounds boneless, center-cut pork loin roast

2 pounds asparagus spears

1 cup cherry tomatoes, halved

DIRECTIONS

1   Preheat the oven to 375 degrees.

2   Place the olive oil in a casserole dish.

3   Mix the thyme, Parmesan cheese, and a little salt and pepper together in a bowl and press the mixture into the pork roast, coating the whole roast evenly.

4   Place the pork, fat cap down, into the casserole dish and roast for 30 minutes.

5   Remove the casserole dish from the oven and remove the pork from the dish to add the asparagus across the bottom of the dish in a single layer. Place the pork onto the asparagus and add the tomatoes to the dish.

6   Roast for another 10 to 15 minutes, depending on the size of the pork roast or until the internal temperature reads 145 degrees on a meat thermometer.

7   Remove the roasted pork from the oven and let sit for about 10 minutes.

8   Slice and serve the pork with the roasted asparagus and the tomatoes.

PER SERVING: *Calories 352; Fat 17g; Cholesterol 168mg; Sodium 571mg; Carbohydrate 8g (Dietary Fiber 4g, Sugar Alcohol 0g); Net Carbohydrate 4g; Protein 42g.*

Creamy Chicken Picatta

PREP TIME: 10 MIN	COOK TIME: 15 MIN	YIELD: 4 SERVINGS

INGREDIENTS

4 tablespoons almond flour

½ cup Parmesan cheese, divided

Salt and pepper

1 large egg

1½ pounds boneless, skinless chicken breasts, halved horizontally and cut in half vertically (to make each breast into 4 pieces)

3 tablespoons salted butter

2 tablespoons minced garlic

1¼ cup chicken broth

3 tablespoons lemon juice

½ cup half-and-half

2 tablespoons capers

DIRECTIONS

1 In a shallow bowl, mix the almond flour and 4 tablespoons of Parmesan cheese, along with a little salt and pepper.

2 Break the egg into a separate shallow bowl.

3 Dip the chicken pieces in the egg bowl first, then dredge them in the almond flour and cheese mixture, and place the coated chicken on a plate.

4 Place the butter in a large skillet over medium-high heat to melt.

5 Add the chicken pieces to the skillet and sear for 4 minutes on each side. The chicken should be nice and browned. Remove the chicken from the pan.

6 Add the garlic to the pan and cook for 1 minute.

7 Pour the chicken broth and lemon juice into the pan and stir. Bring to a simmer.

8 Stir the remaining Parmesan cheese, capers, and half-and-half into the pan.

9 Return the chicken pieces to the skillet and cook for another minute.

10 Serve the chicken immediately and enjoy!

PER SERVING: *Calories 410; Fat 22g; Cholesterol 169mg; Sodium 675mg; Carbohydrate 5g (Dietary Fiber 1g, Sugar Alcohol 0g); Net Carbohydrate 4g; Protein 22g.*

TIP: Enjoy the Creamy Chicken Picatta as is or with your favorite salad or cauliflower rice!

Sausage with Mushroom Onion Gravy

PREP TIME: 5 MIN | COOK TIME: 30 MIN | YIELD: 4 SERVINGS

INGREDIENTS

3 tablespoons olive oil, divided

5 sweet Italian sausage links

3 cups fresh sliced mushrooms

1 cup sliced white onion

1 tablespoon unsalted butter

2 cups beef broth

¼ teaspoon xanthan gum

Salt and pepper to taste

DIRECTIONS

1 Place 2 teaspoons of olive oil in a large skillet and heat over medium heat.

2 Add the sausage links to the skillet and cook for about 10 minutes to cook through. Keep the pan covered as the sausages cook so the juices do not splatter all over. Turn the sausages every 5 minutes to cook evenly.

3 Remove the cooked sausages from the pan and set aside.

4 Add the remaining olive oil, mushrooms, and onion to the skillet and toss. Cook for about 6 minutes to brown the mushrooms and soften the onions.

5 Add the butter and stir to melt.

6 Pour in the beef broth and bring the mixture to a boil.

7 Whisk in the xanthan gum and bring to a boil again to thicken the sauce.

8 Add a little salt and pepper.

9 Add the sausage back to the pan and reheat for about 5 minutes.

10 Serve the sausage and gravy while hot.

PER SERVING: *Calories 576; Fat 51g; Cholesterol 115mg; Sodium 1,487mg; Carbohydrate 5g (Dietary Fiber 1g, Sugar Alcohol 0g); Net Carbohydrate 4g; Protein 23g.*

Chicken Buddha Bowl

PREP TIME: 10 MIN	COOK TIME: 15 MIN	YIELD: 4 SERVINGS

INGREDIENTS

2 tablespoons olive oil, divided

1 pound chicken breast tenders

Salt and pepper

1 red bell pepper, seeds removed, thinly sliced

1 green bell pepper, seeds removed, thinly sliced

1 orange bell pepper, seeds removed, thinly sliced

½ cup sliced red onion

½ cup chicken broth

4 cups grated cauliflower florets or pre-shredded cauliflower rice

1 lime, cut into wedges, for serving

DIRECTIONS

1 Place 1 tablespoon of olive oil in a large skillet and heat over medium-high heat.

2 Sprinkle the chicken breast tenders with a little salt and pepper and then sear in the preheated pan for 4 minutes on each side. Remove the cooked chicken from the pan and set aside.

3 Add the remaining 1 tablespoon of oil to the pan and heat.

4 Add the sliced bell peppers and onions to the skillet and cook for about 5 minutes, stirring occasionally.

5 Remove the sautéed peppers and onion from the skillet.

6 Add the chicken broth and riced cauliflower and cook for 2 minutes to heat.

7 Scoop the rice into four bowls and top each bowl with the pepper and onion mixture and the seared chicken.

8 Serve with lime wedges and enjoy while hot.

PER SERVING: *Calories 447; Fat 28g; Cholesterol 47mg; Sodium 794mg; Carbohydrate 30g (Dietary Fiber 6g, Sugar Alcohol 0g); Net Carbohydrate 24g; Protein 20g.*

Zoodles with Beef Bolognese

PREP TIME: 5 MIN	COOK TIME: 35 MIN	YIELD: 2 SERVINGS

INGREDIENTS

1 pound 80/20 ground beef

8 cloves garlic, chopped, divided

4 cups tomato puree

1 tablespoon chopped fresh basil

1 teaspoon dried oregano

Salt and pepper to taste

3 tablespoons unsalted butter

2 tablespoons olive oil

3 large zucchinis, spiralized into noodles

¼ cup grated Parmesan cheese

DIRECTIONS

1 Place the ground beef in a pot and cook over medium-high heat, breaking up the meat as it cooks to make fine crumbles.

2 Once browned, remove the meat from the pan and set aside.

3 Add half of the garlic to the same pot with the leftover beef grease. Sauté for 1 minute.

4 Add the tomato puree to the pot and stir. Add 1 cup of water and bring the sauce to a simmer. Let the sauce cook for about 10 minutes.

5 Add the cooked ground beef back to the sauce and cook for another 10 minutes, simmering over low heat.

6 Stir the basil into the sauce and season with oregano, salt and pepper. Reduce the heat to low and let simmer.

7 In a separate pot, melt the butter and olive oil over medium heat. Add the rest of the garlic and sauté for 2 minutes.

8 Add the zoodles to the pot and toss. Cook the zoodles in the garlic butter for 5 minutes.

9 Add the Parmesan cheese and toss into the zoodles.

10 Divide the seasoned zoodles among two plates and top each with the Bolognese sauce. Enjoy hot.

PER SERVING: *Calories 1,436; Fat 122g; Cholesterol 217mg; Sodium 1,678mg; Carbohydrate 34g (Dietary Fiber 6g, Sugar Alcohol 0g); Net Carbohydrate 29g; Protein 54g.*

Chunky Guacamole Chicken

PREP TIME: 15 MIN	COOK TIME: 10 MIN	YIELD: 4 SERVINGS

INGREDIENTS

2 tablespoons olive oil

2 tablespoons lime juice

3 tablespoons lime zest

1½ pounds boneless, skinless chicken breast

Guacamole (see the following recipe)

DIRECTIONS

1 In a large bowl, combine the olive oil, lime juice, and lime zest.

2 Add the chicken to the marinade and toss.

3 Cover the bowl and let the chicken marinate for at least 30 minutes or longer in the refrigerator.

4 After the chicken has marinated, preheat a grill or pan to medium-high heat. Grill the chicken for 5 minutes on each side. Discard any extra marinade.

5 While the chicken is cooking, make the guacamole (see the following recipe).

6 Scoop the guacamole over the grilled lime chicken breasts and enjoy while warm.

Guacamole

INGREDIENTS

2 large avocados, peeled, pitted, and chopped

2 tablespoons lime juice

¼ cup chopped cilantro

½ cup chopped red onion

½ cup chopped tomato

Salt and pepper to taste

DIRECTIONS

Combine the avocado, lime juice, cilantro, red onion, and tomato in a large bowl. Stir together with a fork, letting the avocado mash slightly. Add a little salt and pepper.

PER SERVING: *Calories 441; Fat 26g; Cholesterol 124mg; Sodium 86mg; Carbohydrate 16g (Dietary Fiber 8g, Sugar Alcohol 3g); Net Carbohydrate 5g; Protein 41g.*

Meatball Stew with Brussels Sprouts

PREP TIME: 10 MIN	COOK TIME: 26 MIN	YIELD: 4 SERVINGS

INGREDIENTS

1 pound 80/20 ground beef

1 teaspoon minced garlic

1 tablespoon chopped basil

½ cup chopped bacon

4 cups Brussels sprouts, quartered

2 shallots, finely chopped

6 cups beef broth

½ cup heavy cream

Salt and pepper to taste

DIRECTIONS

1 In a large bowl, mix the ground beef, garlic, and basil. Scoop tablespoon-sized balls and roll them between your palms. Set the meatballs aside.

2 Place the chopped bacon in a skillet and sauté over medium heat. Cook for about 5 minutes or until the bacon begins to crisp. Remove the bacon and set aside.

3 Add the meatballs to the hot bacon oil and sear for about 6 minutes, rotating them in the pan until they're brown on all sides. The meatballs will not be cooked but just browned on the outside. Remove them from the pan and set aside.

4 Add the Brussels sprouts and shallots to the pan of bacon grease and sauté. Cook for 5 minutes to soften and brown the Brussels sprouts.

5 Add the beef broth to the pan and put the meatballs and bacon back into the pan. Bring the liquid to a simmer and cook for 10 minutes.

6 Add the heavy cream and stir.

7 Season with salt and pepper and divide the meatball stew among four bowls.

PER SERVING: *Calories 522; Fat 38g; Cholesterol 130mg; Sodium 1,589mg; Carbohydrate 15g (Dietary Fiber 5g, Sugar Alcohol 0g); Net Carbohydrate 10g; Protein 31g.*

Keto Bacon Cheeseburger

PREP TIME: 10 MIN	COOK TIME: 10 MIN	YIELD: 4 SERVINGS

INGREDIENTS

½ cup finely chopped onion

1 pound 85/15 ground beef

1 large egg

½ cup almond flour

Salt and pepper

8 slices cooked bacon, halved

4 slices cheddar cheese

8 butter lettuce leaves

1 tomato, sliced

DIRECTIONS

1 Place the onion, ground beef, egg, almond flour, and a little salt and pepper in a large bowl. Mix the ingredients together with your hands and then divide the meat into four balls. Form ¼-inch-thick patties.

2 Heat a large, cast-iron skillet over medium-high heat.

3 Add the burger patties to the skillet and cook for about 4 minutes on each side for a medium burger.

4 Turn the heat off under the skillet and place four bacon halves on each burger. Place a piece of cheese across the bacon on each burger.

5 Cover the pan and let sit for a minute to melt the cheese.

6 Place each burger on a piece of butter lettuce, add some tomato slices on top, and then top the burger with a second piece of lettuce.

7 Enjoy while hot.

PER SERVING: *Calories 600; Fat 47g; Cholesterol 167mg; Sodium 548mg; Carbohydrate 7g (Dietary Fiber 2g, Sugar Alcohol 0g); Net Carbohydrate 4g; Protein 37g.*

Tomato Basil Chicken

PREP TIME: 35 MIN	COOK TIME: 35 MIN	YIELD: 4 SERVINGS

INGREDIENTS

2 pounds boneless, skinless chicken breasts, cut in half lengthwise

2 tablespoons olive oil

2 teaspoons garlic powder

1 teaspoon Italian seasoning

2 large tomatoes, sliced

4 tablespoons fresh chopped basil

2 cups shredded mozzarella cheese

Salt and pepper

DIRECTIONS

1 In a large bowl, toss the chicken breasts with olive oil, garlic powder, and Italian seasoning. Cover and let sit to marinate in the refrigerator about 20 minutes.

2 Preheat the oven to 425 degrees and spray a casserole dish with cooking spray.

3 Place the marinated chicken in the prepared casserole dish, arranging it in a single layer across the pan.

4 Spread the tomato slices over the chicken and sprinkle the basil over the tomatoes.

5 Cover the chicken and tomatoes with the mozzarella.

6 Sprinkle with a little salt and pepper.

7 Bake in the oven for 35 minutes or until the internal temperature of the chicken is 165 degrees. If the cheese starts to brown too much but the chicken is not yet fully cooked, loosely cover the casserole dish with aluminum foil and continue baking until the chicken is done.

8 Enjoy the chicken while hot!

PER SERVING: *Calories 480; Fat 21g; Cholesterol 194mg; Sodium 400mg; Carbohydrate 7g (Dietary Fiber 1g, Sugar Alcohol 0g); Net Carbohydrate 6g; Protein 62g.*

Rosemary Steak and Brussels Sprouts

| PREP TIME: 5 MIN | COOK TIME: 24 MIN | YIELD: 2 SERVINGS |

INGREDIENTS

2 tablespoons unsalted butter, divided

½ pound Brussels sprouts, halved

½ teaspoon salt

¼ teaspoon ground black pepper

1 teaspoon chopped dried rosemary

1 pound of rib-eye steaks (about 2 steaks)

DIRECTIONS

1 Place 1 tablespoon of butter in a large skillet and heat over medium-high.

2 Add the Brussels sprouts, cut side down, and sear for 12 minutes, tossing after 7 minutes of searing. Remove the Brussels sprouts from the pan and set aside.

3 Place the salt, pepper, and rosemary in a small bowl and mix.

4 Rub the spice mix all over the steaks and let sit for 5 minutes.

5 Place the remaining 1 tablespoon of butter in the same skillet.

6 Add the seasoned steaks to the skillet and sear for about 3 minutes on each side for a medium-rare steak.

7 Serve the hot steak with the seared Brussels sprouts while hot.

PER SERVING: *Calories 682; Fat 41g; Cholesterol 120mg; Sodium 82mg; Carbohydrate 10g (Dietary Fiber 4g, Sugar Alcohol 0g); Net Carbohydrate 6g; Protein 67g.*

Chakhokhbili — Georgian Chicken Stew

INGREDIENTS

2½ pounds chicken thighs, skin on and bone in

Salt and pepper

¼ cup olive oil

½ cup chopped onion

½ cup chopped red bell pepper

1 (28-ounce) can San Marzano tomatoes, chopped

2 jalapeños, diced

½ cup fresh chopped cilantro

1 tablespoon minced garlic

DIRECTIONS

1 Sprinkle the chicken thighs with salt and pepper.

2 Pour the olive oil in a large pot and heat over medium-high heat.

3 Add the seasoned chicken to the pot and sear for 5 minutes. Flip and sear the other side for 3 more minutes. Remove the browned chicken from the pan and set aside.

4 Add the onion and bell pepper to the pan and cook for about 3 minutes, occasionally stirring, to soften the veggies.

5 Add the tomatoes with the canned juices to the pot and bring to a simmer. Cover the pot with a lid, lower the heat to medium, and simmer for 10 minutes.

6 Add the chicken back to the pot, cover, and cook over medium-low heat for 30 minutes.

7 Add the jalapeños, cilantro, and garlic to the pot and stir. Cook for 2 more minutes, then divide into bowls and enjoy hot.

PER SERVING: *Calories 404; Fat 30g; Cholesterol 278mg; Sodium 388mg; Carbohydrate 7g (Dietary Fiber 1g, Sugar Alcohol 0g); Net Carbohydrate 5g; Protein 25g.*

3

Exploring Vegetarian Keto

IN THIS PART . . .

Enjoy a variety of low-carb vegetarian breakfasts.

Make mouth-watering keto vegetarian appetizers.

Keep things simple with keto vegetarian lunches.

Try a variety of flavorful low-carb vegetarian dinners.

Chapter **16**

Vegetarian Breakfasts

A vegetarian diet and a keto diet can go hand-in-hand. The keto diet does not need to revolve around meat or animal products. As with any diet, a good breakfast sets the tone for the entire day. Sticking to your keto diet while meeting your vegetarian needs begins at the breakfast table.

Eggs are a big part of a vegetarian keto diet because they are high in fat and contain a good amount of protein. Be sure to look for local, pasture-raised eggs, which have more omega-3 fatty acids; higher levels of vitamins D, E, and A; and less cholesterol. Chickens on a local farm are more likely to be raised in a humane, animal-friendly way, which is important to many of us, especially those who stick to vegetarian diets due to concern for animals. Farm chickens are happy chickens!

Don't worry, though, eggs are not the only thing you can have for a keto vegetarian breakfast. Pancakes, scones, and even a keto bagel are on our list as well. The recipes in this chapter show you how to create unique and tasty foods that fuel you with fat and keep you full all morning long. Make one of these recipes and you'll be ready for the day.

Berry Noatmeal

PREP TIME: 20 MIN | **COOK TIME: 7 MIN** | **YIELD: 4 SERVINGS**

INGREDIENTS

1 cup sliced, chopped almonds

½ cup unsweetened coconut flakes

½ cup chopped pecans

½ cup raw sunflower seeds

½ cup ground flaxseeds

1 teaspoon raspberry extract

2 tablespoons powdered erythritol

¼ cup unsweetened cocoa powder

2 cups almond milk, divided

1 cup mixed berries, for serving

DIRECTIONS

1 Preheat the oven to 350 degrees and line a rimmed baking sheet with aluminum foil.

2 Spread the almonds, coconut flakes, pecans, and sunflower seeds on the lined baking sheet. Bake for 5 minutes to toast.

3 Place the toasted nut mixture into a food processor along with the flaxseeds, raspberry extract, erythritol, and cocoa powder. Pulse until finely ground.

4 Scoop ¼ cup of the blended mixture and pour into a microwave-safe bowl. Stir in ½ cup almond milk. Microwave on high for 2 minutes and stir well. Repeat this step three more times.

5 Add another ¼ cup of the blended mixture and stir into the noatmeal.

6 Top the noatmeal with the berries and enjoy!

PER SERVING: *Calories 509; Fat 45g; Cholesterol 0mg; Sodium 82mg; Carbohydrate 27g (Dietary Fiber 13g, Sugar Alcohol 0g); Net Carbohydrate 8g; Protein 16g.*

Spinach Feta Egg Muffins

INGREDIENTS

1 cup fresh chopped spinach

½ cup feta cheese crumbles

¼ cup chopped sundried tomatoes

6 large eggs

¼ teaspoon garlic powder

¼ teaspoon salt

¼ teaspoon ground black pepper

DIRECTIONS

1 Preheat the oven to 350 degrees. Grease a muffin pan with cooking spray or butter.

2 Divide the spinach, feta, and sundried tomatoes between six of the greased muffin cups.

3 Whisk the eggs with the garlic powder, salt and pepper, then pour the egg into each muffin cup, pouring the eggs over the veggies and cheese until the muffin cup is about three-fourths full.

4 Bake the egg muffins for 20 minutes, until the eggs are set completely.

5 Serve warm or store in the fridge for up to three days.

PER SERVING: *Calories 102; Fat 7g; Cholesterol 257mg; Sodium 277mg; Carbohydrate 2g (Dietary Fiber 0g, Sugar Alcohol 0g); Net Carbohydrate 2g; Protein 8g.*

Keto Almond Butter Pancakes

PREP TIME: 5 MIN	COOK TIME: 15 MIN	YIELD: 6 SERVINGS

INGREDIENTS

1 cup almond flour

¼ cup coconut flour

3 tablespoons keto protein powder

½ teaspoon baking soda

½ cup almond butter

⅔ cup unsweetened almond milk

2 large eggs

¼ teaspoon cinnamon

Low-carb pancake syrup, for serving

DIRECTIONS

1 Place all ingredients in a blender and puree until the batter is nice and smooth. It may be a little thick, in which case, add a teaspoon more almond milk at a time to get it to a batter-like consistency.

2 Heat a large nonstick skillet over medium heat. Grease the pan with butter.

3 Scoop the pancake batter into the hot skillet, making ¼-cup pancakes. You may have to cook them in batches.

4 Cook for about 3 to 4 minutes until the top of the pancake is bubbling and the bottom is set. Flip the pancakes and cook for another 3 minutes.

5 Remove the pancakes from the skillet and enjoy while warm! Top with low-carb pancake syrup for an extra treat.

PER SERVING: *Calories 310; Fat 23g; Cholesterol 81mg; Sodium 297mg; Carbohydrate 11g (Dietary Fiber 6g, Sugar Alcohol 0g); Net Carbohydrate 5g; Protein 18g.*

Cheesy Keto Bagel with Cream Cheese

PREP TIME: 10 MIN	COOK TIME: 20 MIN	YIELD: 6 SERVINGS

INGREDIENTS

½ cup shredded cheddar cheese

½ cup shredded mozzarella cheese

½ cup grated Parmesan cheese

2 large eggs

1 tablespoon sesame seeds

6 tablespoons cream cheese, divided

DIRECTIONS

1 Preheat the oven to 375 degrees.

2 Whisk the cheddar, mozzarella, and Parmesan cheeses together with the eggs in a bowl.

3 Divide the cheesy egg mixture into six pieces, scooping and pressing the dough into a doughnut pan.

4 Sprinkle the sesame seeds over the top of the dough in the doughnut pan.

5 Bake for 20 minutes. The cheese should be completely melted and have a golden-brown top crust.

6 Let the bagels cool in the pan. Then unmold them, slather 1 tablespoon of cream cheese on each bagel, and enjoy!

PER SERVING: *Calories 165; Fat 13g; Cholesterol 135mg; Sodium 384mg; Carbohydrate 2g (Dietary Fiber 0g, Sugar Alcohol 0g); Net Carbohydrate 2g; Protein 10g.*

Two-Minute Microwave Omelet

PREP TIME: 2 MIN | COOK TIME: 2 MIN | YIELD: 1 SERVING

INGREDIENTS

2 large eggs

1 tablespoon milk

1 tablespoon shredded cheddar cheese

2 cherry tomatoes, quartered

1 tablespoon fresh chopped basil

Salt and pepper

DIRECTIONS

1 Place the eggs and milk in a bowl. Whisk them together well.

2 Add the remaining ingredients and stir with a fork.

3 Spray a microwave-safe soup or cereal bowl with cooking spray and add the mixture to it. Microwave the eggs on medium for 60 seconds. The eggs will begin to look set. Microwave again for another 30 seconds or continue to microwave in 30-second increments until the center of the omelet is completely set.

4 Let the omelet cool slightly and then enjoy.

PER SERVING: *Calories 194; Fat 14g; Cholesterol 84mg; Sodium 58mg; Carbohydrate 2g (Dietary Fiber 1g, Sugar Alcohol 0g); Net Carbohydrate 2g; Protein 15g.*

Chocolate Protein Pancakes

PREP TIME: 5 MIN	COOK TIME: 10 MIN	YIELD: 2 SERVINGS

INGREDIENTS

½ cup egg white protein powder

½ cup almond flour

¼ cup unsweetened cocoa powder

¼ cup powdered erythritol

1 teaspoon baking powder

4 large eggs

⅓ cup unsweetened coconut milk

2 tablespoons coconut oil, melted

1 teaspoon vanilla extract

¼ teaspoon salt

Low-carb pancake syrup, fresh fruit, or powdered erythritol, for topping

DIRECTIONS

1 Place all the ingredients (except toppings) into a large bowl and use a whisk to mix until very smooth.

2 Heat a large nonstick skillet over medium–low heat. Spray the pan with cooking spray.

3 Scoop ¼ cup of the batter into the pan per pancake. Add as many pancakes as you can, without letting them touch, and cook for 3 minutes. Flip and cook the pancake for another 2 minutes.

4 Move the pancake to a plate and repeat the cooking process with the remaining pancakes.

5 Enjoy while warm with pancake syrup, some fresh fruit, or powdered erythritol dusted on top.

PER SERVING: *Calories 548; Fat 38g; Cholesterol 160mg; Sodium 327mg; Carbohydrate 40g (Dietary Fiber 9g, Sugar Alcohol 24g); Net Carbohydrate 8g; Protein 40g.*

Veggie Breakfast Bake

PREP TIME: 15 MIN	COOK TIME: 1 HOUR	YIELD: 8 SERVINGS

INGREDIENTS

2 cups broccoli florets

1 chopped red bell pepper

½ cup chopped white onion

Salt and pepper

3 tablespoons olive oil, divided

2 cups baby spinach, lightly packed

1 cup chopped tomatoes

12 large eggs

½ cup whole milk

1 teaspoon Italian seasoning

1 cup shredded cheddar cheese

DIRECTIONS

1 Preheat the oven to 400 degrees. Grease a 9-x-13-inch casserole dish and a baking sheet.

2 Spread the broccoli florets, bell pepper, and onion on the greased baking sheet. Sprinkle with some salt and pepper and drizzle with 2 tablespoons of olive oil.

3 Toss the spinach and tomatoes in the remaining 1 tablespoon of olive oil; then add them to the greased baking sheet with the other veggies.

4 Roast the veggies for 20 minutes.

5 While the veggies bake, whisk together the eggs, milk, Italian seasoning, and a little salt and pepper.

6 Place the roasted veggies into the greased casserole dish. Pour the egg mixture over the veggies and then sprinkle the top of the casserole with the cheese.

7 Lower the oven temperature to 300 degrees and bake the casserole for 35 to 40 minutes or until the center of the casserole no longer jiggles. Slice and serve immediately.

PER SERVING: *Calories 223; Fat 17g; Cholesterol 512mg; Sodium 405mg; Carbohydrate 5g (Dietary Fiber 2g, Sugar Alcohol 0g); Net Carbohydrate 4g; Protein 13g.*

Keto Berry Scones

PREP TIME: 10 MIN | **COOK TIME: 35 MIN** | **YIELD: 4 SERVINGS**

INGREDIENTS

¾ cup blueberries, raspberries, chopped strawberries or mixed

½ cup granular erythritol, divided

⅓ cup coconut flour

1½ cups almond flour

2 teaspoons baking powder

⅓ cup heavy cream

3 tablespoons unsalted butter, melted

2 large eggs, separated

Sliced almonds, for topping (optional)

DIRECTIONS

1 Preheat the oven to 350 degrees. Line a baking sheet with parchment paper

2 Place the berries in a small pot with ¼ cup of the erythritol. Bring to a boil and let simmer for 10 minutes to thicken. Set aside to cool.

3 In a large bowl, mix the coconut flour, almond flour, remaining ¼ cup of erythritol, and baking powder.

4 Stir the heavy cream, melted butter, and egg yolks into the dry ingredients and knead into a smooth dough.

5 Scoop the dough into ¼-cup flat-ish circles and place them on the parchment-lined baking sheet. Space the scones about 2 inches apart.

6 Indent the center of each scone and scoop ½ tablespoon of the cooked berries into the center of each scone.

7 Brush the edges and tops of the scones with the egg whites. Sprinkle with some sliced almonds, if desired.

8 Bake for 25 minutes or until golden brown. Enjoy warm.

PER SERVING: Calories 483; Fat 40g; Cholesterol 129mg; Sodium 241mg; Carbohydrate 44g (Dietary Fiber 9g, Sugar Alcohol 24g); Net Carbohydrate 11g; Protein 14g.

Chapter **17**

Vegetarian Appetizers

E veryone loves a good appetizer. Having easy recipes to make quick, delicious bites is essential for variety and for helping you stay on track with your diet when cravings hit.

Not only do meal appetizers help placate your need for food, but they also help boost any macro needs you may have. If your fat intake is down for the day, you can make a few fat bombs to enjoy. If you feel like you need a few more veggies in your diet, broccoli bites may be your answer.

In this chapter, we provide a good starting point for vegetarian keto appetizers. You can serve many of these alongside your favorite meals. Make a tray of Spinach Mozzarella Mushrooms to pass around at a party with an Italian dinner on the menu. Matcha Energy Balls are a great precursor to a keto Chinese food dinner.

You'll find a wide array of flavors in this section, and there's something for everyone. Non-vegetarian, non-keto followers will enjoy these apps and snacks as well. They'll never even know that they are diet-friendly foods!

Broccoli Bites

PREP TIME: 10 MIN	COOK TIME: 10 MIN	YIELD: 4 SERVINGS (2 BITES EACH)

INGREDIENTS

½ pound broccoli florets

1 cup shredded cheddar cheese

2 large eggs

3 tablespoons almond flour

½ teaspoon garlic powder

¼ cup olive oil

DIRECTIONS

1 Place the broccoli in a microwave-safe bowl and pour 3 tablespoons of water over the top. Cover with a plate and microwave on high for 3 to 4 minutes, until broccoli is tender. Drain any extra water. Let the broccoli cool.

2 Place the broccoli, cheese, eggs, almond flour, and garlic powder in a food processor and pulse until a thick dough forms.

3 Heat the olive oil in a medium skillet over medium heat.

4 Scoop the dough into eight equal-sized balls (about 2 tablespoons each) and drop the balls into the hot oil.

5 Fry the broccoli for 5 minutes, flipping throughout until all sides are golden brown.

6 Enjoy while hot.

PER SERVING: *Calories 311; Fat 28g; Cholesterol 109mg; Sodium 227mg; Carbohydrate 5g (Dietary Fiber 3g, Sugar Alcohol 0g); Net Carbohydrate 2g; Protein 12g.*

Cheesy Baked Tomatoes

PREP TIME: 10 MIN	COOK TIME: 10 MIN	YIELD:8 SERVINGS (2 TOMATO HALVES EACH)

INGREDIENTS

8 large Roma tomatoes, cut in half

1 cup shredded mozzarella cheese

1 cup shredded Parmesan cheese

½ cup fresh chopped basil

¼ cup fresh chopped parsley

2 tablespoons olive oil

DIRECTIONS

1 Preheat the oven to 400 degrees and line a 9-x-13-inch glass baking dish with aluminum foil.

2 Place the halved tomatoes in the lined dish, cut side facing up and scoop out the centers along with the seeds to make room for the cheese.

3 In a small bowl, combine together the remaining ingredients.

4 Pile the cheese mixture into each tomato.

5 Drizzle the tomatoes with the olive oil and then place the dish in the oven.

6 Roast the tomatoes for about 10 minutes, browning the cheese and letting the tomatoes get nice and soft.

7 Serve immediately.

PER SERVING: Calories 114; Fat 8g; Cholesterol 17mg; Sodium 188mg; Carbohydrate 3g (Dietary Fiber 1g, Sugar Alcohol 0g); Net Carbohydrate 3g; Protein 7g.

Spinach Mozzarella Mushrooms

PREP TIME: 15 MIN	COOK TIME: 25 MIN	YIELD: 4 SERVINGS (5 MUSHROOMS EACH)

INGREDIENTS

1 tablespoon olive oil

10 ounces frozen spinach, thawed, squeezed dry

8 ounces cream cheese (1 cup)

½ cup shredded Parmesan cheese

¾ cup finely shredded mozzarella cheese, divided

1½ teaspoons minced garlic

Salt and pepper

20 cremini mushrooms, cleaned, stems removed

DIRECTIONS

1   Preheat the oven to 400 degrees. Line a baking sheet with aluminum foil and grease it with the olive oil.

2   Roughly chop the thawed, dried spinach and place it in a large bowl. Add the cream cheese, Parmesan cheese, ½ cup of shredded mozzarella, garlic, and a sprinkle of salt and pepper. Stir the ingredients together well.

3   Place the mushrooms on the prepared baking sheet, hollowed side up. The mushrooms should look like little bowls.

4   Scoop the spinach and cheese mixture into each mushroom cap, filling each to a little over the top.

5   Sprinkle the mushrooms with the remaining ¼ cup of mozzarella cheese.

6   Bake the mushrooms in the oven for about 20 to 25 minutes or until the tops are golden brown.

7   Serve immediately and enjoy!

PER SERVING: *Calories 425; Fat 21g; Cholesterol 92mg; Sodium 766mg; Carbohydrate 12g (Dietary Fiber 3g, Sugar Alcohol 0g); Net Carbohydrate 9g; Protein 21g.*

No-Bake Peanut Butter Balls

PREP TIME: 10 MIN	COOK TIME: NONE	YIELD: 4 SERVINGS (3 BALLS EACH)

INGREDIENTS

2 tablespoons unsweetened shredded coconut

½ cup smooth peanut butter

2 tablespoons coconut flour

2 tablespoons powdered erythritol

2 tablespoons low-carb pancake syrup

¼ cup unsweetened shredded coconut

1 tablespoon almond milk

DIRECTIONS

1 Place the shredded coconut in a food processor and pulse until it is fine crumbs. Pour into a shallow bowl and set aside.

2 Place the remaining ingredients into a bowl and stir until a thick dough forms.

3 Scoop the dough into 12 equal-sized portions and roll with your hands into smooth balls.

4 Roll the balls in the coconut crumbs, then place them on a plate. Store the peanut butter balls in the fridge or enjoy them right away.

PER SERVING: *Calories 266; Fat 22g; Cholesterol 0mg; Sodium 7mg; Carbohydrate 21g (Dietary Fiber 6g, Sugar Alcohol 7g); Net Carbohydrate 7g; Protein 8g.*

Matcha Energy Balls

PREP TIME: 10 MIN	COOK TIME: NONE	YIELD: 8 SERVINGS (1 BALL EACH)

INGREDIENTS

½ cup shredded coconut

½ cup almond flour

2 tablespoons chia seeds

1 tablespoon pure matcha tea powder plus extra for serving

½ cup peanut butter

1 tablespoon unsweetened almond milk

3 tablespoons low carb pancake syrup

Powered erythritol, for serving (optional)

DIRECTIONS

1 Combine all the ingredients (except the extra matcha and erythritol) in a large bowl and mix well until a thick dough forms.

2 Place the mixture in the fridge for 30 minutes to chill.

3 Scoop the mixture into 2 tablespoon-sized balls and roll between your palms until smooth.

4 Roll each ball in a little extra matcha powder and powdered erythritol, if desired.

5 Store in the fridge until ready to enjoy!

PER SERVING: *Calories 193; Fat 16g; Cholesterol 0mg; Sodium 7mg; Carbohydrate 10g (Dietary Fiber 5g, Sugar Alcohol 1g); Net Carbohydrate 4g; Protein 6g.*

Pepper and Cheese Mushrooms

PREP TIME: 15 MIN	COOK TIME: 30 MIN	YIELD: 4 SERVINGS (5 MUSHROOMS EACH)

INGREDIENTS

20 baby Bella mushrooms, rubbed clean with a paper towel

½ cup diced red bell pepper

1 teaspoon olive oil

1 teaspoon minced garlic

8 ounces cream cheese (1 cup)

½ cup shredded Parmesan cheese

1 teaspoon Italian seasoning

Salt and pepper to taste

DIRECTIONS

1 Preheat the oven to 350 degrees and line a baking sheet with aluminum foil.

2 Remove the stems from the mushrooms and set aside.

3 Place the mushrooms on the prepared baking sheet with the stems removed, hollowed side up. The mushrooms should look like little bowls.

4 Chop the mushroom stems and add them to a large skillet with bell pepper and olive oil. Heat the pan over medium–high heat and cook for about 5 minutes, stirring occasionally.

5 Add the garlic to the pan and stir again. Cook for 2 more minutes; then remove the pan from the heat and set aside to cool.

6 Stir the cream cheese, Parmesan, Italian seasoning, and salt and pepper together in a large bowl.

7 Add the cooled mushroom and pepper mix to the cream cheese and stir well.

8 Scoop the mix into each mushroom cap, stuffing them as full as possible.

9 Bake the stuffed mushrooms for about 20 minutes or until the tops begin to brown slightly. Enjoy warm.

PER SERVING: *Calories 347; Fat 28g; Cholesterol 83mg; Sodium 613mg; Carbohydrate 8g (Dietary Fiber 2g, Sugar Alcohol 0g); Net Carbohydrate 6g; Protein 17g.*

Chapter **18**

Vegetarian Lunches

L unch can be one of the hardest meals of the day. Many of us eat lunch outside of our home. Whether you are out and about on the weekend or at work during the week, you may need to pack your lunch in advance and take it with you. Finding keto vegetarian lunches at restaurants, delis, or take-out joints can be quite tricky, so having meals that travel well is essential. You don't want to ruin your keto diet with a bad lunch!

There are plenty of recipes in this section that you can use for meal prep. Chocolate Peanut Butter Chia Bowls are great for making at the beginning of the week, as are our Bell Pepper Egg Cups. Microwave muffins are a fantastic quick meal that you can put together in a matter of minutes, giving you a healthy, vegetarian meal with little prep or cooking time.

Be sure to plan your lunch so you don't have to skip this essential meal. Having a good keto lunch gives you a boost of energy to power you through the rest of the workday. There are plenty of sweet and savory lunch ideas here that give you the right balance of keto macros while also checking all your boxes for flavor, simplicity, and vegetarian ingredients.

Chocolate Peanut Butter Chia Bowl

PREP TIME: 25 MIN | COOK TIME: NONE | YIELD: 2 SERVINGS

INGREDIENTS

4 tablespoons peanut butter

1½ cups almond milk

1 tablespoon unsweetened cocoa powder

½ teaspoon ground cinnamon

½ cup ice

1 teaspoon vanilla extract

3 tablespoons chia seeds, divided

1 tablespoon hemp seeds, divided

½ cup blueberries, divided

DIRECTIONS

1 Place the peanut butter, almond milk, cocoa powder, cinnamon, ice, and vanilla extract in a blender and puree until very smooth.

2 Add 2 tablespoons of the chia seeds and blend again.

3 Pour the mixture into two bowls and top each with 1½ teaspoons of the remaining chia seeds, 1½ teaspoons of hemp seeds, and ¼ cup of blueberries. Let cool in the refrigerator for at least 20 minutes to thicken up.

4 Serve while cold.

PER SERVING: *Calories 382; Fat 26g; Cholesterol 0mg; Sodium 70mg; Carbohydrate 25g (Dietary Fiber 14g, Sugar Alcohol 0g); Net Carbohydrate 12g; Protein 13g.*

Bell Pepper Egg Cups

PREP TIME: 10 MIN	COOK TIME: 25 MIN	YIELD: 4 SERVINGS

INGREDIENTS

2 small red or green bell peppers

4 large eggs

Salt and pepper

1 tablespoon fresh chopped parsley

DIRECTIONS

1 Preheat the oven to 350 degrees.

2 Cut each pepper in half from top to bottom and remove the seeds.

3 Rest the peppers, cut side up, on the baking sheet.

4 Crack each egg into the hollow pepper.

5 Sprinkle each with salt and pepper.

6 Bake the pepper eggs for 25 minutes. The yolk should still be slightly runny, but the whites should be firm.

7 Sprinkle the parsley over the eggs and then enjoy immediately.

PER SERVING: *Calories 339; Fat 4g; Cholesterol 160mg; Sodium 65mg; Carbohydrate 5g (Dietary Fiber 2g, Sugar Alcohol 0g); Net Carbohydrate 3g; Protein 6g.*

Peanut Butter Microwave Muffin

PREP TIME: 5 MIN	COOK TIME: 2 MIN	YIELD: 1 SERVING

INGREDIENTS

1½ tablespoons coconut oil

1 tablespoon brown sugar erythritol

1 egg white

2½ tablespoons creamy peanut butter

2 tablespoons almond flour

1 tablespoon coconut flour

¼ teaspoon xanthan gum

¼ teaspoon baking powder

1 tablespoon Lily's low-carb chocolate chips

DIRECTIONS

1 In a small bowl, mix the coconut oil, erythritol, and egg white together.

2 Stir in the peanut butter and mix until smooth.

3 Add the remaining ingredients to the batter and stir until combined.

4 Scoop the muffin batter into a greased, microwave-safe mug.

5 Microwave on high for about 75 seconds. The center of the muffin should spring back to the touch.

6 Let cool for about 5 minutes, and then enjoy right out of the mug!

PER SERVING: *Calories 582; Fat 52g; Cholesterol 0mg; Sodium 170mg; Carbohydrate 35g (Dietary Fiber 10g, Sugar Alcohol 14g); Net Carbohydrate 12g; Protein 17g.*

TIP: You can find Lily's low-carb chocolate chips in most large supermarkets in the baking aisle.

Cauliflower Pancakes

PREP TIME: 10 MIN	COOK TIME: 15 MIN	YIELD: 6 SERVINGS

INGREDIENTS

2 (10-ounce) boxes frozen cauliflower florets

2 large eggs

¾ cup shredded cheddar cheese

¼ cup chopped green onions

¼ cup coconut flour

½ teaspoon cayenne pepper

2 tablespoons olive oil

½ cup sour cream, for serving

DIRECTIONS

1 Bring a large pot of water to a boil and cook the cauliflower florets for 5 minutes. Drain the water and then place the cauliflower in a large bowl.

2 Mash the cauliflower into a chunky puree.

3 Stir in the eggs, cheese, onions, coconut flour, and cayenne.

4 Pour the olive oil into a large skillet and heat over medium-high heat.

5 Scoop ¼ cup of the cauliflower batter into the hot oil, fitting as many small pancakes into the pan as you can. (You will likely have to cook the pancakes in batches.)

6 Fry the pancakes for 3 minutes; flip and fry for another 3 minutes.

7 Remove the pancakes from the skillet and place them on a paper towel to drain.

8 Serve with sour cream on top.

PER SERVING: *Calories 195; Fat 15g; Cholesterol 79mg; Sodium 154mg; Carbohydrate 8g (Dietary Fiber 3g, Sugar Alcohol 0g); Net Carbohydrate 4g; Protein 8g.*

Super Green Smoothie Bowl

PREP TIME: 5 MIN	COOK TIME: NONE	YIELD: 2 SERVINGS

INGREDIENTS

1 large avocado

1½ cups unsweetened almond milk

1 cup baby spinach, lightly packed

1 cup plain, unsweetened yogurt

¼ cup low-carb pancake syrup

1 tablespoon coconut oil

1 cup ice

1 teaspoon vanilla extract

2 teaspoons chia seeds, divided

¼ cup sliced almonds, divided

½ cup fresh blueberries, divided

2 tablespoons sunflower seeds, divided

DIRECTIONS

1 Place the avocado, almond milk, baby spinach, yogurt, pancake syrup, coconut oil, ice, and vanilla extract in a blender and puree until very smooth.

2 Pour the smoothie into two bowls and top each with 1 teaspoon of chia seeds, 2 tablespoons of sliced almonds, ¼ cup of blueberries, and 1 tablespoon of sunflower seeds. Enjoy cold.

PER SERVING: *Calories 524; Fat 39g; Cholesterol 17mg; Sodium 250mg; Carbohydrate 43g (Dietary Fiber 22g, Sugar Alcohol 5g); Net Carbohydrate 16g; Protein 14g.*

Peanut Berry Smoothie Bowl

PREP TIME: 5 MIN	COOK TIME: NONE	YIELD: 2 SERVINGS

INGREDIENTS

½ cup canned coconut milk

1 scoop (30g) low-carb protein powder

2 tablespoons peanut butter

1 tablespoon low-carb pancake syrup

1 teaspoon vanilla extract

½ teaspoon cinnamon

1 cup ice

½ cup fresh blueberries, divided

2 teaspoons chia seeds, divided

¼ cup chopped, salted peanuts, divided

DIRECTIONS

1 Place the coconut milk, protein powder, peanut butter, pancake syrup, vanilla extract, cinnamon, and ice in a blender and puree until very smooth. Pour into two bowls.

2 Top each bowl with ¼ cup of blueberries, 1 teaspoon of chia seeds, and 2 tablespoons of chopped peanuts. Enjoy while cold.

PER SERVING: *Calories 324; Fat 20g; Cholesterol 1mg; Sodium 99mg; Carbohydrate 18g (Dietary Fiber 7g, Sugar Alcohol 1g); Net Carbohydrate 10g; Protein 23g.*

Cheesy Cauliflower Muffins

PREP TIME: 10 MIN	COOK TIME: 25 MIN	YIELD: 8 MUFFINS

INGREDIENTS

2½ cups riced cauliflower (about ½ head of cauliflower riced)

2 large eggs

1 cup shredded cheddar cheese

¼ cup almond flour

½ teaspoon salt

½ teaspoon baking powder

¼ teaspoon garlic powder

DIRECTIONS

1 Preheat the oven to 375 degrees and grease eight wells of a muffin pan with nonstick spray.

2 Mix all the ingredients together in a large bowl until a thick batter forms.

3 Scoop the mixture into the prepared muffin cups so they are about two-thirds full.

4 Bake the muffins for about 20 to 25 minutes, until they are completely set and no longer look wet.

5 Let the muffins cool completely before removing them from the pan to enjoy.

PER SERVING: *Calories 220; Fat 17g; Cholesterol 54mg; Sodium 180mg; Carbohydrate 5g (Dietary Fiber 2g, Sugar Alcohol 0g); Net Carbohydrate 3g; Protein 12g.*

Three Cheese Frittata

PREP TIME: 5 MIN	COOK TIME: 15 MIN	YIELD: 6 SERVINGS

INGREDIENTS

1 tablespoon olive oil

1 large leek, halved, chopped, and rinsed

6 large eggs

¼ cup heavy cream

1 teaspoon salt

¼ teaspoon ground black pepper

½ cup crumbled goat cheese

½ cup shredded cheddar cheese

½ cup grated Parmesan cheese

DIRECTIONS

1 Preheat the oven to 400 degrees.

2 In a large oven-safe skillet, heat the olive oil over medium-high heat.

3 Add the sliced leeks to the skillet and sauté for about 5 minutes, stirring occasionally. Remove the pan from the heat.

4 In a medium bowl, whisk together the eggs, heavy cream, salt and pepper.

5 Stir all the cheeses into the egg mixture and then pour into the pan over the sautéed leeks.

6 Place the skillet into the oven and bake for 10 minutes or until the eggs are completely set.

7 Remove the pan from the oven and let the frittata cool for about 5 minutes; then slice and serve.

PER SERVING: *Calories 229; Fat 18g; Cholesterol 197mg; Sodium 271mg; Carbohydrate 3g (Dietary Fiber 0g, Sugar Alcohol 0g); Net Carbohydrate 3g; Protein 14g.*

Chapter **19**

Vegetarian Dinners

t's the end of the day and you are ready for a delicious, complete meal. Of course, you also want to stick to your keto diet and your vegetarian preferences as well. If this sounds familiar, you have come to the right place. This chapter is packed with incredible vegetarian keto dinners that help you complete a perfect day of low-carb eating.

It isn't too hard to meet your fat macros when on a vegetarian diet. The harder macro to hit is the protein. When you are on a vegetarian diet, you skip the big pieces of protein-filled meat and opt to find protein in plant-based sources. Nuts, low-carb grains, and tofu are delicious ingredients that are high in protein. Cooking with dairy is another way to add protein to a vegetarian dinner. Luckily, we keto dieters also love cheese! It's one of the best vegetarian keto ingredients we can think of.

All our vegetarian keto dinners focus on unique flavors as well as balanced ingredients. You get your keto fats and your vegetarian proteins without any worry of carbs. Even if you're not on a vegetarian diet, we recommend giving a few of these recipes a try. They're a refreshing break from heavy, meat-packed dinners.

Cauliflower Crust Pizza

PREP TIME: 10 MIN	COOK TIME: 30 MIN	YIELD: 4 SERVINGS

INGREDIENTS

1 head cauliflower, chopped

2 large eggs, beaten

1½ cups shredded mozzarella, divided

1 tablespoon Italian seasoning

¼ teaspoon ground black pepper

½ cup Rao's pizza sauce

½ cup shredded Parmesan cheese

1 tomato, sliced

¼ cup chopped fresh basil

DIRECTIONS

1 Preheat the oven to 425 degrees and line a baking sheet with parchment paper.

2 Place the cauliflower florets in a food processor and pulse until they are finely ground and look like rice.

3 Pour the cauliflower into a microwave-safe bowl, cover, and microwave on high for 5 minutes. Let cool, then place the cauliflower in a dish towel, wrap it tightly in the towel, and squeeze, getting out as much moisture as possible.

4 Place the dried cauliflower in a bowl and stir in the eggs, ½ cup mozzarella, Italian seasoning, and pepper.

5 Spread the cauliflower mixture on the parchment-lined baking sheet, making it into a 14-inch circle.

6 Bake the crust for 20 minutes, so it is golden brown.

7 Spread the sauce over the crust, then sprinkle with the remaining mozzarella, Parmesan cheese, and tomato slices.

8 Bake for another 3 minutes to melt the cheeses.

9 Remove the pizza from the oven, sprinkle with the fresh basil, and then enjoy!

PER SERVING: *Calories 232; Fat 13g; Cholesterol 111mg; Sodium 488mg; Carbohydrate 12g (Dietary Fiber 4g, Sugar Alcohol 0g); Net Carbohydrate 9g; Protein 18g.*

Thai Curry Soup

PREP TIME: 10 MIN   **COOK TIME: 30 MIN**   **YIELD: 4 SERVINGS**

INGREDIENTS

1 (8-ounce) block extra-firm tofu, pressed and cut into cubes

3 tablespoons soy sauce

2 tablespoons coconut oil

2 red bell peppers, sliced

1 small bok choy, cut into strips (4–5 cups)

½ cup chopped onion

1 tablespoon fresh grated ginger

2 cloves garlic, minced

1 teaspoon lime juice

1 green chili pepper, chopped

¼ teaspoon ground cumin

¼ teaspoon ground cayenne pepper

1½ cups canned coconut milk, unsweetened

1 cup vegetable broth

1 tablespoon granular erythritol

1 handful roughly chopped cilantro

DIRECTIONS

1 In a medium bowl, combine cubed tofu and soy sauce. Mix until the tofu absorbs the soy sauce.

2 Pour the coconut oil in a large pan and heat over medium-high heat. Add tofu mixture and sauté until evenly browned on all or most sides.

3 Move the tofu to the side of the pan and add the pepper slices and sauté for 2 minutes.

4 Add the bok choy to the pan and cook for another 2 minutes. Then remove the tofu and veggies from the pan and set aside.

5 Place the onion in the pan and cook for 2 minutes.

6 Add the ginger, garlic, lime juice, green chili, cumin, and cayenne. Stir and cook for 4 minutes.

7 Add the peppers and bok choy back into the pan along with the coconut milk, vegetable broth, and erythritol. Stir and cook over low heat for 15 minutes.

8 Divide among four bowls, garnish with chopped cilantro and enjoy. You can also serve the curry over cauliflower rice for an even more filling meal.

PER SERVING: *Calories 333; Fat 30g; Cholesterol 0mg; Sodium 792mg; Carbohydrate 16g (Dietary Fiber 3g, Sugar Alcohol 3g); Net Carbohydrate 10g; Protein 10g.*

Cauliflower Parmesan and Zoodles with Tomato Sauce

PREP TIME: 15 MIN	COOK TIME: 25 MIN	YIELD: 4 SERVINGS

INGREDIENTS

1 large head cauliflower, thickly sliced into 1-inch steaks

1 tablespoon olive oil

1 teaspoon Italian seasoning

½ teaspoon salt

¼ teaspoon ground black pepper

2 cups Rao's tomato sauce, divided

½ pound shredded mozzarella cheese

1 tablespoon unsalted butter

1 teaspoon minced garlic

⅓ cup almond flour

2 large zucchinis, ends trimmed

¼ cup grated Parmesan cheese

DIRECTIONS

1   Preheat the oven to 425 degrees.

2   Place the cauliflower steaks on a rimmed baking sheet.

3   Use a pastry brush to brush the olive oil on the cauliflower. Sprinkle with the Italian seasoning, salt and pepper; then place in the oven to roast for 15 minutes.

4   Remove the baking sheet from the oven and pour 1 cup of tomato sauce over the cauliflower slices.

5   Sprinkle the mozzarella over each cauliflower steak, then bake for another 10 minutes or until the cheese is bubbly.

6   While the cauliflower is roasting, melt the butter in a small skillet and add the garlic. Sauté to brown the garlic, then stir in the almond flour to make garlic "breadcrumbs."

7   Use a spiralizer to cut the zucchini into noodles.

8   Fill a small pot with water and bring it to a boil. Add the zoodles and cook for 2 minutes. Drain the noodles.

9   Divide the cauliflower and zoodles among four plates.

10 Sprinkle the "breadcrumbs" over the cooked cauliflower along with the Parmesan cheese. Top the zoodles with the remaining tomato sauce and enjoy!

PER SERVING: *Calories 465; Fat 31g; Cholesterol 49mg; Sodium 862mg; Carbohydrate 19g (Dietary Fiber 7g, Sugar Alcohol 0g); Net Carbohydrate 19g; Protein 24g.*

Egg Shakshuka

PREP TIME: 5 MIN	COOK TIME: 22 MIN	YIELD: 4 SERVINGS

INGREDIENTS

2 tablespoons olive oil

1 cup chopped red bell pepper

½ cup chopped onion

1 tablespoon minced garlic

1 tablespoon paprika

1 teaspoon ground cumin

¼ teaspoon chili powder

1 (28-ounce) can diced tomatoes

½ teaspoon salt

¼ teaspoon ground black pepper

8 large eggs

½ cup chopped cilantro

½ cup chopped parsley

Crumbled feta cheese, for serving (optional)

DIRECTIONS

1 Pour the olive oil in a large skillet and heat over medium heat.

2 Add the bell peppers and onion to the pan and cook for 5 minutes.

3 Add the garlic, paprika, cumin, and chili powder and stir. Cook for 1 more minute.

4 Add the tomatoes and juice into the pan. Add the salt and pepper; then bring the mixture to a simmer for 5 to 10 minutes.

5 Use a spoon to make eight wells in the sauce and then crack one egg into each well.

6 Cover the pan and cook for 6 minutes. The eggs should be set. Cook a little longer for a firmer yolk.

7 Sprinkle the cilantro, parsley, and feta cheese (if desired) over the pan and then divide among four plates.

PER SERVING: Calories 257; Fat 15g; Cholesterol 320mg; Sodium 341mg; Carbohydrate 16g (Dietary Fiber 4g, Sugar Alcohol 0g); Net Carbohydrate 12g; Protein 14g.

Cauliflower Fried Rice Bowl

| PREP TIME: 5 MIN | COOK TIME: 17 MIN | YIELD: 4 SERVINGS |

INGREDIENTS

1 tablespoon olive oil

1 garlic clove, minced

½ cup chopped white onion

½ pound firm tofu, cubed

1 cup chopped red bell pepper

1 medium zucchini, chopped

3 tablespoons coconut aminos

1 tablespoon lime juice

5 cups cauliflower florets

1 cup shredded white cheddar cheese

2 large eggs

DIRECTIONS

1 Pour the olive oil in a pan on medium-high heat.

2 Add the garlic and onion and sauté for 2 minutes.

3 Add the cubed tofu to the pan and sauté for 3 to 4 minutes until the tofu is golden brown.

4 Add the chopped peppers, zucchini, coconut aminos, and lime juice to the pan and cook while stirring for 5 minutes.

5 Place the cauliflower florets in a food processor and pulse the cauliflower until small rice-like pieces are formed.

6 Add the cauliflower to the pan and cook while stirring for another 5 minutes.

7 Stir in the cheese to melt.

8 Whisk the eggs in a small bowl and pour them into the pan. Stir constantly and cook until scrambled, about 1 minute.

9 Divide the cauliflower stir-fry into four bowls and enjoy!

PER SERVING: *Calories 330; Fat 20g; Cholesterol 109mg; Sodium 460mg; Carbohydrate 11g (Dietary Fiber 4g, Sugar Alcohol 0g); Net Carbohydrate 11g; Protein 21g.*

Stuffed Zucchini with Cheesy Rice

PREP TIME: 20 MIN	COOK TIME: 20 MIN	YIELD: 4 SERVINGS

INGREDIENTS

Cheesy Rice:

6 cups cauliflower rice

1 cup shredded cheddar cheese

½ cup sour cream

1 teaspoon onion powder

2 teaspoons garlic powder

Zucchini Boats:

¼ cup unsalted butter

2 cloves garlic, minced

1 cup heavy cream

1 cup Parmesan cheese

¼ teaspoon salt

¼ teaspoon ground black pepper

4 medium zucchinis

1 cup chopped tomatoes, divided

½ cup white cheddar cheese

DIRECTIONS

1 Preheat the oven to 400 degrees.

2 Start by making the cheesy rice. Combine all the ingredients in a medium-sized bowl and then spread the mixture in a greased 9-x-13-inch casserole dish.

3 Bake the cheesy rice in the oven for 20 minutes. It should be bubbling around the edges, and the cheese on top should be melted.

4 While the cheesy rice is cooking, make the zucchini boats. Melt the butter in a small pot over medium heat. Add the garlic and sauté for 2 to 3 minutes.

5 Add the heavy cream and bring to a simmer. Cook for 5 minutes.

6 Stir in the Parmesan cheese, salt and pepper. Set the sauce aside to cool.

7 Cut each zucchini in half lengthwise. Scoop the center out of each zucchini, turning them into boats.

8 Place the zucchini halves on an oiled, rimmed baking sheet.

9 Scoop 2 tablespoons of the chopped tomatoes into each zucchini boat.

10 Fill the boats with the sauce, pouring the sauce over the tomatoes.

11 Sprinkle the cheddar cheese over the zucchini boats and then bake for about 10 minutes to melt the cheese. It should be bubbling and golden brown.

12 Serve zucchini boats alongside the warm cheesy rice.

PER SERVING: *Calories 741; Fat 63g; Cholesterol 190mg; Sodium 794mg; Carbohydrate 20g (Dietary Fiber 6g, Sugar Alcohol 0g); Net Carbohydrate 14g; Protein 26g.*

Cheesy Cauliflower Muffins

PREP TIME: 10 MIN | **COOK TIME: 25 MIN** | **YIELD: 8 MUFFINS**

INGREDIENTS

2½ cups riced cauliflower (about ½ head cauliflower, riced)

2 large eggs, whipped

1 cup shredded cheddar cheese

¼ cup almond flour

½ teaspoon salt

½ teaspoon baking powder

¼ teaspoon garlic powder

DIRECTIONS

1 Preheat the oven to 375 degrees and spray eight wells of a muffin pan with cooking spray.

2 Combine all the ingredients together in a large bowl until a thick batter forms.

3 Scoop the mixture into the muffin wells so they are about two-thirds full.

4 Bake the muffins for about 20 to 25 minutes, until they are completely set and no longer look wet.

5 Let the muffins cool completely before removing them from the pan to enjoy.

PER SERVING: *Calories 220; Fat 17g; Cholesterol 109mg; Sodium 340mg; Carbohydrate 5g (Dietary Fiber 2g, Sugar Alcohol 0g); Net Carbohydrate 3g; Protein 12g.*

Pesto Zoodles

INGREDIENTS

1 teaspoon garlic powder

3 tablespoons almond flour

¼ teaspoon salt plus more for the pesto

¼ teaspoon ground black pepper plus more for the pesto

1 pound extra-firm tofu, cut into 1-inch cubes

3 tablespoons olive oil

2 large zucchinis, ends trimmed

2 cups fresh packed basil

2 cloves garlic

⅓ cup olive oil

⅓ cup pine nuts

½ cup grated Parmesan cheese

2 teaspoons lemon juice

DIRECTIONS

1 Start by making the fried tofu. Mix the garlic powder, almond flour, salt and pepper in a medium-sized bowl.

2 Toss the tofu cubes in the flour mixture, coating completely.

3 Heat the olive oil in a medium-sized skillet over medium-high heat.

4 Add the tofu to the pan and fry for 3 minutes. Flip each cube individually and fry for another 3 minutes.

5 Once the tofu is golden brown, remove and set it aside to start making the zoodles.

6 Use a spiralizer to turn the zucchini into noodles. Sauté the zoodles, in the same skillet used for the tofu, on medium heat for about 2 to 3 minutes. Transfer the sautéed zoodles into a large bowl.

7 Make a pesto by placing the basil, garlic, olive oil, pine nuts, Parmesan cheese, lemon juice, and a sprinkle of salt and pepper to a food processor. Pulse until all the ingredients are smooth. Be sure to wipe down the sides of the food processor to get all the pieces well blended.

8 Add the pesto to the bowl with the zoodles. Toss the zoodles in the pesto and then divide them among four bowls. Top with the fried tofu and sprinkle with a little extra Parmesan cheese. Enjoy!

PER SERVING: *Calories 531; Fat 48g; Cholesterol 10mg; Sodium 134mg; Carbohydrate 11g (Dietary Fiber 4g, Sugar Alcohol 0g); Net Carbohydrate 11g; Protein 20g.*

TIP: If you do not have a spiralizer, use a peeler to cut the zucchini into strips and a knife to turn the strips into long noodles.

Broccoli Calzone

PREP TIME: 20 MIN   COOK TIME: 20 MIN   YIELD: 2 SERVINGS

INGREDIENTS

1 cup almond flour

3 tablespoons coconut flour

2 teaspoons xanthan gum

1 teaspoon baking powder

½ teaspoon salt

1 tablespoon apple cider vinegar

2 large eggs

1 cup grated mozzarella cheese

½ cup goat cheese

½ cup ricotta cheese

1 cup small, chopped broccoli florets

3 tablespoons minced garlic

¼ cup fresh chopped basil

1 cup Rao's tomato sauce, for dipping

DIRECTIONS

1   Start by making the keto calzone dough. Place the almond flour, coconut flour, xanthan gum, baking powder, and salt in a food processor and pulse together.

2   Add the vinegar and pulse again.

3   Add one egg and 1 tablespoon of water and run the food processor until a dough forms. Wrap the sticky dough in plastic wrap and set aside to rest.

4   Preheat the oven to 400 degrees and line a baking sheet with parchment paper.

5   Next, make the filling. In a medium bowl, mix the mozzarella, goat, and ricotta cheeses; broccoli; garlic; and basil together.

6   Divide the keto dough into two pieces and roll each ball between two pieces of parchment paper until they are each about ⅛-inch thick.

7   Scoop about ½ cup of filling into the center of each dough circle and then fold the circle in half, enclosing the filling completely.

8   Pinch the edges of each calzone together. Place the calzones on the prepared baking sheet.

9   Whisk the remaining egg in a small bowl. Brush the tops of each calzone with the whisked egg and then bake for 20 minutes. The calzones should be golden brown.

10   Serve while warm with a side of tomato sauce for dipping.

PER SERVING: *Calories 458; Fat 33g; Cholesterol 120mg; Sodium 616mg; Carbohydrate 17g (Dietary Fiber 7g, Sugar Alcohol 0g); Net Carbohydrate 11g; Protein 24g.*

4

Maximizing Your Meals with Air Fryers, Slow Cookers, and Meal Prep

IN THIS PART . . .

Discover air frying recipes that will make your mouth water.

Enjoy the simplicity of Instant Pot and slow cooker recipes.

· Save time and money with delicious meal-prep recipes.

Chapter **20**

Air Fryer Recipes

You already know that we love keto, but another one of our kitchen loves is the air fryer. The air fryer is such a useful tool that can help you make incredible snacks, side dishes, breakfasts, and even full dinners. We wanted to combine our kitchen passions and create keto-friendly, air fryer meals. Each of these recipes is easy, quick, and surprisingly healthy for "fried" food.

Air fryers can help make foods crispy and crunchy as if they were deep fried. However, you only need to use a small amount of oil rather than a big pot of fryer oil. While oils and fats are okay on the keto diet, deep frying can still be wasteful. You need to use so much oil to fry small quantities of food, and this oil typically gets thrown away. The oil you use to air fry foods is all eaten rather than disposed of.

We also love the air fryer because it is so easy to use. You can cook a complete keto meal in the air fryer in a matter of minutes. We know that cooking all your keto foods can be time consuming, especially when you are still getting adjusted to keto recipes. A nice air fryer meal can be a refreshing change of pace.

REMEMBER

Try not to pile foods into your air fryer basket (or tray) but rather spread every-thing out in a single layer. Air fryers work by circulating hot air around the basket of ingredients. If the basket is packed too tightly, the air can't move around the food properly. This prevents your food from getting crispy and cooked. One layer of food with space between items is best, or you can create two layers that are separated using an air fryer rack, which is an accessory you can purchase if your air fryer doesn't have one.

Burger Fat Bombs

PREP TIME: 10 MIN	COOK TIME: 15 MIN	YIELD: 6 SERVINGS

INGREDIENTS

1½ pounds 85/15 ground beef

⅓ cup almond flour

1 large egg

2 tablespoons chopped parsley

1 teaspoon Italian seasoning

1 tablespoon melted butter

Salt and pepper to taste

DIRECTIONS

1 Preheat the air fryer to 400 degrees.

2 Mix all the ingredients together in a large bowl.

3 Scoop into two to three tablespoon-sized meatballs.

4 Place the meatballs on the air fryer basket and cook for 15 minutes.

5 Skewer each burger ball with a toothpick and enjoy.

PER SERVING: *Calories 352; Fat 28g; Cholesterol 112mg; Sodium 86mg; Carbohydrate 2g (Dietary Fiber 1g, Sugar Alcohol 0g); Net Carbohydrate 1g; Protein 22g.*

Seared Scallops and Asparagus

PREP TIME: 5 MIN	COOK TIME: 6 MIN	YIELD: 2 SERVINGS

INGREDIENTS

½ teaspoon salt

¼ teaspoon ground black pepper

½ teaspoon garlic powder

2 tablespoons olive oil

1 pound large sea scallops

1 pound asparagus, ends trimmed

3 tablespoons butter

1 teaspoon minced garlic

1 tablespoon lemon juice

DIRECTIONS

1 Preheat the air fryer to 400 degrees.

2 Place the salt and pepper, garlic powder, and olive oil in a large bowl and mix them together.

3 Add the scallops and asparagus spears to the bowl and toss, coating the asparagus and scallops in the seasoning.

4 Spread the asparagus and scallops on the air fryer basket, making one single layer.

5 Cook in the air fryer for 6 minutes, flipping them midway through.

6 In the meantime, make the garlic butter. Place the butter, garlic, and lemon juice in a small, microwave-safe bowl and microwave on high for about 30 seconds to melt the butter.

7 Divide the asparagus and scallops between two plates and drizzle both with the melted garlic butter. Enjoy while warm.

PER SERVING: *Calories 526; Fat 33g; Cholesterol 117mg; Sodium 332mg; Carbohydrate 16g (Dietary Fiber 5g, Sugar Alcohol 0g); Net Carbohydrate 12g; Protein 40g.*

Pork Tenderloin and Almond Flour Brussels Sprouts

PREP TIME: 15 MIN	COOK TIME: 25 MIN	YIELD: 4 SERVINGS

INGREDIENTS

1 tablespoon smoked paprika

1 tablespoon granular erythritol

1¾ teaspoons salt, divided

½ teaspoon onion powder

¾ teaspoon ground black pepper, divided

1½ pounds pork tenderloin

2 tablespoons olive oil, divided

½ teaspoon garlic powder

½ cup almond flour

½ cup grated Parmesan cheese

1 pound Brussels sprouts, halved

DIRECTIONS

1 Preheat the air fryer to 400 degrees.

2 Place the paprika, erythritol, 1½ teaspoons of salt and pepper and ½ teaspoon of onion powder in a small bowl and stir.

3 Rub the pork tenderloin with 1 tablespoon of olive oil and then rub the spice mix over the entire outside of the pork tenderloin. Place on the air fryer basket.

4 Air fry the pork tenderloin for 10 minutes. While the pork is frying, start making the Brussels sprouts.

5 Place the garlic powder, the remaining 1/4 teaspoon each of salt and pepper, almond flour, and Parmesan cheese in a large bowl and stir.

6 Toss the Brussels sprouts in the remaining 1 tablespoon of olive oil and then toss them in the almond flour mix, coating them as much as possible in the seasoning.

7 Add the Brussels sprouts to the air fryer basket, spreading them around the pork tenderloin.

8 Return the basket to the air fryer to cook for another 15 minutes. The sprouts should be nice and brown, and the pork should be crisp on top and have an internal temperature of 150 degrees.

9 Slice the pork tenderloin and serve it alongside the crispy Brussels sprouts.

PER SERVING: Calories 458; Fat 24g; Cholesterol 120mg; Sodium 1,185mg; Carbohydrate 18g (Dietary Fiber 7g, Sugar Alcohol 3g); Net Carbohydrate 8g; Protein 46g.

Air Fryer Chicken and Veggies

PREP TIME: 10 MIN	COOK TIME: 27 MIN	YIELD: 4 SERVINGS

INGREDIENTS

½ teaspoon garlic powder

½ teaspoon chili powder

½ teaspoon salt

½ teaspoon ground black pepper

1 tablespoon Italian seasoning

2 tablespoons olive oil, divided

1 pound chicken thighs, bone in and skin on

1 cup broccoli florets

1 medium zucchini, sliced

1 cup cherry tomatoes

1 cup chopped red or green bell pepper

1 red onion, chopped

1 tablespoon chopped garlic

DIRECTIONS

1 Preheat the air fryer to 400 degrees and spray your air fryer basket with cooking spray.

2 Place the garlic powder, chili powder, salt and pepper, and Italian seasoning in a small bowl; then stir in 1 tablespoon of olive oil. In a large bowl, combine half the seasoning mixture with the chicken thighs and mix gently until well coated.

3 Place the chicken thighs on the air fryer basket.

4 Cook the chicken thighs in the air fryer for 15 minutes.

5 Place all the remaining ingredients in a large bowl and toss with the leftover spice mixture and the remaining 1 tablespoon of olive oil.

6 Remove the air fryer basket and spread the veggies on the tray along with the half-cooked chicken.

7 Return the basket to the air fryer to cook for another 12 minutes.

8 Divide the chicken and veggies among four plates and enjoy while hot.

PER SERVING: *Calories 362; Fat 26g; Cholesterol 111mg; Sodium 117mg; Carbohydrate 11g (Dietary Fiber 4g, Sugar Alcohol 0g); Net Carbohydrate 7g; Protein 21g.*

NOTE: You may need to air fry the chicken thighs in batches, but the total cook time will increase.

Air Fryer Chicken with Cauliflower Rice

PREP TIME: 15 MIN	COOK TIME: 20 MIN	YIELD: 4 SERVINGS

INGREDIENTS

4 boneless, skinless chicken breasts

½ teaspoon salt plus more for the cauliflower rice

¼ teaspoon ground black pepper plus more for the cauliflower rice

1 teaspoon paprika

½ teaspoon onion powder

½ teaspoon garlic powder

4 tablespoon olive oil

6 cups cauliflower florets

1 onion, chopped

2 tablespoons fresh chopped parsley

2 tablespoons lemon juice

4 cups baby spinach, lightly packed

DIRECTIONS

1 Preheat the air fryer to 375 degrees.

2 Place the chicken breast on a clean work surface, cover with a sheet of plastic wrap to prevent splatter and use a meat mallet or rolling pin to pound it lightly to tenderize the meat.

3 Place the salt and pepper, paprika, onion powder, and garlic powder in a small bowl and stir the seasonings together.

4 Drizzle the chicken with 1 tablespoon of olive oil, then sprinkle the spice mix over the chicken, rubbing the seasonings on both sides of the chicken breasts.

5 Place the seasoned chicken breasts in the air fryer basket and cook for 12 minutes. The internal temperature should be 165 degrees.

6 While the chicken cooks, make the cauliflower rice. Place the cauliflower in a food processor and pulse until it resembles rice.

7 Pour the remaining olive oil in a large skillet and heat over medium-high heat.

8 Add the onion to the pan and sauté for 2 minutes.

9 Add the cauliflower rice to the pan and stir. Cook for another 2 minutes.

(continued)

10 Add the parsley, lemon juice, a little salt and pepper, and spinach to the pan and stir until the spinach has wilted.

11 Divide the cauliflower rice among four plates and serve with the chicken.

PER SERVING: *Calories 389; Fat 18g; Cholesterol 127mg; Sodium 142mg; Carbohydrate 10g (Dietary Fiber 3g, Sugar Alcohol 0g); Net Carbohydrate 7g; Protein 42g.*

Pistachio-Crusted Salmon and Veggies

PREP TIME: 15 MIN	COOK TIME: 15 MIN	YIELD: 4 SERVINGS

INGREDIENTS

4 (6-ounce) salmon filets

Salt and pepper

2 cloves garlic, minced

2 tablespoons olive oil

¼ teaspoon Dijon mustard

3 tablespoons lemon juice

⅔ cup shelled pistachios, finely chopped

2 tablespoons unsalted butter

1½ pounds asparagus

1 cup grape tomatoes, halved

1 teaspoon garlic powder

⅓ cup freshly grated Parmesan cheese

DIRECTIONS

1 Preheat the air fryer to 400 degrees. Spray the air fryer basket with cooking spray.

2 Place the salmon filets on a plate and season with a little salt and pepper.

3 In a small bowl, mix the garlic, olive oil, mustard, and lemon juice. Spread the mixture over each salmon filet.

4 Spread the pistachios over each salmon filet, patting them down as you place them on the fish.

5 Place the filets in the air fryer and cook for 15 minutes.

6 While the fish is cooking, place the butter in a large skillet. Add the asparagus spears and tomatoes cover the pan and cook for 5 minutes.

7 Sprinkle the asparagus and tomatoes with garlic powder and Parmesan cheese, and then divide the veggies among four bowls. Place the cooked pistachio salmon on top of the veggies and enjoy.

PER SERVING: *Calories 64; Fat 47g; Cholesterol 115mg; Sodium 220mg; Carbohydrate 15g (Dietary Fiber 6g, Sugar Alcohol 0g); Net Carbohydrate 9g; Protein 46g.*

Spicy Air Fryer Halloumi Bites

PREP TIME: 5 MIN	COOK TIME: 10 MIN	YIELD: 2 SERVINGS

INGREDIENTS

½ pound halloumi cheese, cut into 1-inch cubes

1 tablespoon olive oil

¼ teaspoon ground red pepper flakes

¼ teaspoon garlic powder

DIRECTIONS

1 Preheat the air fryer to 375 degrees.

2 Place the halloumi cubes in a large bowl and toss with the olive oil, red pepper flakes, and garlic powder.

3 Place the halloumi cubes in a single layer in the air fryer basket.

4 Cook for 7 to 10 minutes until the edges of the cheese are golden brown and crispy.

5 Enjoy hot.

PER SERVING: *Calories 426; Fat 39g; Cholesterol 81mg; Sodium 1,203mg; Carbohydrate 0g (Dietary Fiber 0g, Sugar Alcohol 0g); Net Carbohydrate 0g; Protein 24g.*

Caprese Stuffed Chicken

PREP TIME: 10 MIN	COOK TIME: 15 MIN	YIELD: 4 SERVINGS

INGREDIENTS

4 boneless, skinless chicken breasts

½ cup baby spinach, finely chopped, divided

½ cup fresh basil leaves, finely chopped, divided

1 cup sundried tomatoes in oil, divided

4 slices fresh mozzarella cheese

1½ teaspoons Italian seasoning

¼ teaspoon salt

¼ teaspoon ground black pepper

DIRECTIONS

1 Preheat the air fryer to 400 degrees. Spray your air fryer rack with cooking spray.

2 Place the chicken breast on a clean work surface and cut a pocket into each chicken breast, cutting it three-fourths of the way through.

3 Stuff each chicken breast with 2 tablespoons each of spinach and basil, ¼ cup of sundried tomatoes, and one slice of mozzarella cheese.

4 Secure each chicken breast closed using toothpicks, then place them on the air fryer basket.

5 Lightly spray the chicken with olive oil cooking spray. Sprinkle with the Italian seasoning, salt and pepper.

6 Cook the chicken in the air fryer for 15 minutes or until fully done, having an internal temperature of 165 degrees.

7 Let the chicken cool for about 5 minutes and enjoy while warm.

PER SERVING: *Calories 360; Fat 15g; Cholesterol 152mg; Sodium 355mg; Carbohydrate 8g (Dietary Fiber 2g, Sugar Alcohol 0g); Net Carbohydrate 6g; Protein 47g.*

Zucchini Pizza Bites

PREP TIME: 10 MIN	COOK TIME: 10 MIN	YIELD: 2 SERVINGS

INGREDIENTS

1 medium zucchini

2 tablespoons olive oil

1 teaspoon dried basil

¼ teaspoon salt

¼ teaspoon ground black pepper

4 tablespoons tomato sauce

8 slices pepperoni

8 tablespoons mozzarella cheese

DIRECTIONS

1 Preheat the air fryer to 400 degrees.

2 Slice the zucchini on a diagonal into eight ¾-inch-thick ovals. Place the slices in a large bowl.

3 Add the olive oil, basil, salt and pepper to the bowl and toss the zucchini slices, coating them in the seasoned olive oil completely.

4 Place the oiled zucchini on the air fryer basket.

5 Top each zucchini slice with 1½ teaspoons of tomato sauce, 1 slice of pepperoni, and a tablespoon of mozzarella cheese.

6 Cook the zucchini for 10 minutes. The cheese should be melted and golden brown.

7 Enjoy while hot!

PER SERVING: *Calories 262; Fat 23g; Cholesterol 22mg; Sodium 381mg; Carbohydrate 6g (Dietary Fiber 1g, Sugar Alcohol 0g); Net Carbohydrate 5g; Protein 8g.*

Jalapeño Stuffed Mini Meatloaf with Green Salad

PREP TIME: 25 MIN	COOK TIME: 15 MIN	YIELD: 4 SERVINGS

INGREDIENTS

6 ounces cream cheese (¾ cup), softened

½ cup shredded cheddar cheese

8 jalapeños, tops cut off and seeds removed

1 pound 85/15 ground beef

1 large egg

1 tablespoon coconut flour

1 teaspoon garlic powder

1 teaspoon salt

¼ teaspoon ground black pepper

4 strips bacon, cut in half

8 cups mixed greens

¼ cup olive oil

2 tablespoons lemon juice

2 teaspoons Dijon mustard

DIRECTIONS

1 Preheat the air fryer to 400 degrees and line your air fryer basket with air fryer parchment paper.

2 In a small bowl, mix the cream cheese and cheddar cheese.

3 Stuff the jalapeños with the cream cheese mixture, packing each jalapeño as full as possible.

4 In a medium bowl, mix the ground beef, egg, coconut flour, garlic powder, salt and pepper.

5 Take about ½ cup of the meat mixture and pat it in your hand to look like a disc. Place a stuffed jalapeño in the center and then enclose the jalapeño in the meat mix. Wrap the jalapeño completely in meat, rolling the little meatloaf in your hand to make it nicely shaped. Repeat, wrapping all the jalapeños in the ground beef.

6 Wrap each mini meatloaf in a half strip of bacon and place it in the parchment-lined air fryer basket.

7 Cook for 15 minutes. The bacon should be crispy, and the meatloaf cooked.

8 While the meatloaves are air-frying, place the mixed greens in a large bowl; then add the olive oil, lemon juice, and mustard. Toss the lettuce in the dressing completely, then divide it among four plates.

9 Place two mini meatloaves on each plate and enjoy.

PER SERVING: *Calories 754; Fat 65g; Cholesterol 196mg; Sodium 550mg; Carbohydrate 9g (Dietary Fiber 3g, Sugar Alcohol 0g); Net Carbohydrate 7g; Protein 32g.*

Greek Stuffed Peppers

PREP TIME: 10 MIN	COOK TIME: 20 MIN	YIELD: 2 SERVINGS

INGREDIENTS

2 red or green bell peppers

1 tablespoon olive oil

¼ cup chopped onion

¼ pound ground beef

¼ pound 80/20 ground lamb

1 teaspoon dried oregano

1 teaspoon dried basil

¼ teaspoon salt

8 ounces diced tomatoes (roughly 1 cup)

1 cup feta cheese

DIRECTIONS

1 Preheat the air fryer to 400 degrees. Spray the air fryer basket with cooking spray.

2 Cut the bell peppers in half and scoop out and discard the seeds. Place the pepper halves in the air fryer basket, open side up.

3 Pour the olive oil into a large pan and heat over medium-high heat. Add the onion and sauté for 1 minute.

4 Add the ground beef and ground lamb to the pan and stir, breaking up the meat as it cooks. Cook the meat for about 6 minutes, so it is still a little pink.

5 Add the oregano, basil, and salt and stir.

6 Add the tomatoes to the pan and stir again.

7 Remove the pan from the heat and stir in the feta cheese.

8 Divide the meat mixture between the peppers, stuffing them so they are overflowing with filling.

9 Cook the peppers in the air fryer for 10 minutes, then serve while hot.

PER SERVING: *Calories 629; Fat 48g; Cholesterol 148mg; Sodium 770mg; Carbohydrate 17g (Dietary Fiber 5g, Sugar Alcohol 0g); Net Carbohydrate 13g; Protein 32g.*

Coconut Shrimp Salad

PREP TIME: 15 MIN	COOK TIME: 10 MIN	YIELD: 4 SERVINGS

INGREDIENTS

¼ cup almond flour

½ teaspoon garlic powder

½ teaspoon salt

2 large eggs

¾ cup unsweetened shredded coconut

1 pound extra-large shrimp, peeled and deveined

½ cup sour cream

2 tablespoons olive oil

¼ cup Dijon mustard

1 tablespoon apple cider vinegar

4 cups mixed greens

DIRECTIONS

1 Preheat the air fryer to 350 degrees. Spray your air fryer basket with cooking spray.

2 Mix the almond flour, garlic powder, and salt in a shallow bowl.

3 Whisk the eggs in a separate bowl.

4 Place the shredded coconut in a third bowl.

5 Dip the shrimp in the almond-flour mixture; then in the egg; and finally, coat it in the coconut. When all the shrimp are coated, place them into the air fryer basket.

6 Cook the coconut shrimp for 10 minutes, flipping halfway through. It should be golden brown and crispy.

7 While the shrimp cooks, whisk the sour cream, olive oil, mustard and vinegar in a large bowl.

8 Add the mixed greens to the bowl and toss the lettuce in the dressing.

9 Divide the greens among four bowls, top the salad with the cooked coconut shrimp, and enjoy.

PER SERVING: *Calories 392; Fat 30g; Cholesterol 238mg; Sodium 882mg; Carbohydrate 13g (Dietary Fiber 5g, Sugar Alcohol 3g); Net Carbohydrate 5g; Protein 23g.*

Bacon-Wrapped Shrimp

PREP TIME: 15 MIN	COOK TIME: 12 MIN	YIELD: 4 SERVINGS

INGREDIENTS

1 teaspoon garlic salt

2 teaspoons chili powder

2 teaspoons coconut aminos

2 tablespoons low-carb pancake syrup

1 pound jumbo shrimp, cooked

10 slices bacon, cut in half

DIRECTIONS

1 Preheat the air fryer to 400 degrees and spray your air fryer basket with cooking spray.

2 In a large bowl, combine the garlic salt, chili powder, coconut aminos, and pancake syrup.

3 Add the shrimp to the bowl and toss to coat the shrimp in the thick sauce.

4 Wrap each seasoned shrimp in a half piece of bacon. When all the shrimp are wrapped, place them in the air fryer basket with the end on the bacon strip down, so it stays securely on the shrimp.

5 Cook for 12 minutes to crisp the bacon, and then enjoy while hot.

PER SERVING: *Calories 262; Fat 13g; Cholesterol 257mg; Sodium 1,720mg; Carbohydrate 7g (Dietary Fiber 3g, Sugar Alcohol 1g); Net Carbohydrate 3g; Protein 29g.*

Bacon Chicken Cheesy Bites

PREP TIME: 10 MIN	COOK TIME: 20 MIN	YIELD: 4 SERVINGS

INGREDIENTS

1 teaspoon smoked paprika

½ teaspoon chili powder

½ teaspoon garlic salt

¼ teaspoon dried thyme

12 boneless, skinless chicken wings

6 slices cheddar cheese, cut in half

12 slices bacon

DIRECTIONS

1 Preheat the air fryer to 400 degrees.

2 Add the paprika, chili powder, garlic salt, and thyme to a small bowl and stir.

3 Sprinkle the seasoning over the wings.

4 Place half a slice of cheese on top of each wing, then wrap each wing with a strip of bacon, enclosing the cheese and chicken wing as much as possible.

5 Place the wrapped chicken wings in the air fryer basket.

6 Cook the wings in the air fryer for 10 minutes; then flip and cook for another 10 minutes.

7 Serve while hot with your favorite keto BBQ sauce.

PER SERVING: *Calories 592; Fat 47g; Cholesterol 228mg; Sodium 812mg; Carbohydrate 2g (Dietary Fiber 0g, Sugar Alcohol 0g); Net Carbohydrate 1g; Protein 40g.*

Parmesan Pork with Crispy Veggies

PREP TIME: 10 MIN	COOK TIME: 25 MIN	YIELD: 2 SERVINGS

INGREDIENTS

Cheese Sauce (see the following recipe)

4 center cut, boneless pork chops

½ teaspoon salt

¼ teaspoon ground black pepper

2 cups pork rind crumbs

⅓ cup grated Parmesan cheese

½ teaspoon garlic powder

½ teaspoon onion powder

¼ teaspoon chili powder

2 large eggs

1 cup broccoli florets

1 cup cauliflower florets

DIRECTIONS

1 Make the cheese sauce (see the following recipe). Set aside.

2 Preheat the air fryer to 400 degrees.

3 Sprinkle the pork chops with the salt and pepper.

4 Place the pork rind crumbs, Parmesan cheese, garlic powder, onion powder, and chili powder in a food processor and pulse together. Pour half the mix into a small bowl and reserve the other half.

5 Whisk one of the eggs in a shallow bowl.

6 Dip the pork chops in the whisked egg and then into the pork rind mixture, coating each pork chop completely in the pork rinds. Place the coated chops on a plate while you prepare the veggies.

7 Whisk the remaining egg in a small bowl and pour the remaining pork rind mixture into another shallow bowl.

8 Toss the broccoli and cauliflower in the egg and then toss it in the pork rind mixture. Spread the coated veggies on the air fryer basket in between the pork chops.

9 Cook the pork chops and veggies for 20 minutes in the air fryer. Everything should be golden brown and crispy.

10 Divide among four plates and pour the cheese sauce over each plate. Enjoy while warm.

Cheese Sauce

INGREDIENTS

4 ounces cream cheese (½ cup)

½ cup unsalted butter

½ cup heavy cream

1 cup mozzarella cheese

DIRECTIONS

1 Place the cream cheese, butter, and heavy cream in a small pot and melt over medium heat.

2 Whisk in the mozzarella cheese until completely melted.

PER SERVING: *Calories 1,327; Fat 136g; Cholesterol 602mg; Sodium 1,189mg; Carbohydrate 7g (Dietary Fiber 1g, Sugar Alcohol 0g); Net Carbohydrate 6g; Protein 136g.*

Italian Chicken and Veggies

PREP TIME: 10 MIN	COOK TIME: 20 MIN	YIELD: 2 SERVINGS

INGREDIENTS

2 boneless, skinless chicken breasts, cut into 1-inch cubes

1 cup broccoli florets

1 cup sliced red or green bell peppers

1 medium zucchini, sliced

1 cup grape tomatoes, quartered

1 small onion, sliced

2 tablespoons olive oil

1 tablespoon Italian seasoning

1 teaspoon smoked paprika

2 teaspoons minced garlic

½ teaspoon salt

¼ teaspoon ground black pepper

DIRECTIONS

1 Preheat the air fryer to 400 degrees.

2 Line the air fryer basket with air fryer parchment paper.

3 Place all the ingredients in a large bowl and toss them together well.

4 Pour the ingredients into the parchment-lined basket and spread flat.

5 Cook in the air fryer for 20 minutes, stirring halfway through.

6 Divide between two plates and enjoy while warm.

PER SERVING: *Calories 404; Fat 19g; Cholesterol 127mg; Sodium 107mg; Carbohydrate 16g (Dietary Fiber 6g, Sugar Alcohol 0g); Net Carbohydrate 10g; Protein 43g.*

Chapter **21**

Instant Pot and Slow Cooker Meals

We don't all have time to prepare a five-course meal every night. Many of us don't even have time to cook a one-course meal. We all lead busy lives, and any dinner shortcuts we can take are always appreciated.

That's where an Instant Pot comes in handy. One-pot and one-pan meals are some of our favorites. We love the simplicity that these meals offer. You can make complete, healthy meals without the mess and hassle of extra bowls and dishes to clean up. Most Instant Pot meals are also super hearty.

Slow cooker meals are also effortless to make. Most of them require dumping all the ingredients into the pot, giving the mix a quick stir, and then coming back hours later to a perfectly cooked meal.

Use our easy, Instant Pot and slow cooker recipes to hit your macro targets, prepare flavorful dinners, and have little to clean up. For the recipes in this chapter, you can use a 5 to 6 quart Instant Pot or slow cooker. Once you start using these appliances, you'll wish every recipe could be made this easily. There's nothing like coming home to the scent of a delicious recipe filling the air and a meal just waiting for you to sit down and eat.

Instant Pot Mushroom Pork Chops

PREP TIME: 10 MIN	COOK TIME: 20 MIN	YIELD: 6 SERVINGS

INGREDIENTS

6 boneless pork chops

¼ teaspoon salt

¼ teaspoon ground black pepper

2 tablespoons olive oil

2 tablespoons unsalted butter

2 cups sliced mushrooms

1 cup heavy cream

2 tablespoons chopped parsley

1 tablespoon fresh chopped thyme

3 tablespoons minced garlic

4 cups broccoli florets

DIRECTIONS

1 Sprinkle the pork chops with the salt and pepper.

2 Set the Instant Pot to sauté, and then add the olive oil and butter.

3 Place the pork chops in the Instant Pot in batches and cook for 1 minute on each side to brown. Remove the pork chops from the pot.

4 Add the mushrooms to the Instant Pot along with the heavy cream and simmer, scraping the bottom of the pot.

5 Return the pork chops to the Instant Pot with the mushrooms and cream. Add the parsley, thyme, and garlic and stir.

6 Cover and seal the Instant Pot and cook on high pressure for 8 minutes. Let the Instant Pot do a natural steam release and then carefully open the lid.

7 Add the broccoli florets to the pan and place the lid back on the pot. Cook on high pressure for 1 more minute.

8 Divide the broccoli and pork chops among six plates and enjoy. You can also place the meal in meal-prep containers and store them in the fridge.

PER SERVING: *Calories 843; Fat 41g; Cholesterol 393mg; Sodium 295mg; Carbohydrate 6g (Dietary Fiber 3g, Sugar Alcohol 0g); Net Carbohydrate 4g; Protein 108g.*

Slow Cooker Chipotle Chicken Soup

PREP TIME: 15 MIN | COOK TIME: 6 HOURS | YIELD: 4 SERVINGS

INGREDIENTS

½ cup chopped onions

4 celery stalks, chopped

1 (14-ounce) can diced tomatoes

2 chipotle chilis in adobo sauce

1 teaspoon chili powder

8 cups chicken broth

½ teaspoon salt

¼ teaspoon ground black pepper

6 large boneless chicken thighs, cubed

1 medium avocado, chopped

DIRECTIONS

1 Place the onions, celery, diced tomatoes, chili peppers, chili powder, chicken broth, salt and pepper to the bowl of the slow cooker and stir.

2 Add the chicken thighs. Cover with the lid.

3 Cook over high heat for 4 to 6 hours.

4 Divide the soup into four bowls and top each bowl with a quarter of the chopped avocado.

PER SERVING: *Calories 502; Fat 21g; Cholesterol 282mg; Sodium 2,236mg; Carbohydrate 15g (Dietary Fiber 6g, Sugar Alcohol 0g); Net Carbohydrate 8g; Protein 63g.*

Slow Cooker Beef and Broccoli

PREP TIME: 15 MIN | **COOK TIME: 8 HOURS** | **YIELD: 8 SERVINGS**

INGREDIENTS

2 pounds beef chuck, cut into 1-inch cubes

1½ cup beef broth

¾ cup tamari sauce

¼ tablespoons sesame oil

6 cloves garlic, minced

4 cups broccoli florets

1 cup chopped scallions

1 red bell pepper, sliced

1 green bell pepper, sliced

1 tablespoon coconut flour

1 tablespoon sesame seeds

DIRECTIONS

1 In a large pan on high heat, brown the beef until browned on all sides. Place the beef cubes, beef broth, tamari sauce, sesame oil, and garlic into a slow cooker and cook on high for 6 to 8 hours.

2 In the last 30 minutes of cooking, add the broccoli, scallions, and sliced peppers to the slow cooker. Additionally, in a small bowl, mix the coconut flour and 2 tablespoons of water. Stir into the slow cooker and cover with the lid.

3 Divide between eight meal-prep containers and enjoy throughout the week. Garnish with sesame seeds before serving.

PER SERVING: *Calories 265; Fat 14g; Cholesterol 73mg; Sodium 860mg; Carbohydrate 8g (Dietary Fiber 3g, Sugar Alcohol 0g); Net Carbohydrate 5g; Protein 29g.*

Instant Pot Keto Chili

INGREDIENTS

2 tablespoons olive oil

1 cup chopped white onions

¼ cup minced garlic

2 pounds 80/20 ground beef

1 (28-ounce) can diced tomatoes

1 (6-ounce) can tomato paste

1 (4-ounce) can green chiles

¼ cup chili powder

2 tablespoons ground cumin

1 tablespoon dried oregano

2 teaspoons salt

1 teaspoon ground black pepper

2 bay leaves

DIRECTIONS

1 Place the olive oil into your Instant Pot and press sauté.

2 Add the onions and sauté for 2 minutes.

3 Add the garlic and ground beef and sauté for 3 more minutes to brown the beef. Break it up with your spoon as it cooks to make small pieces.

4 Add all the remaining ingredients to the Instant Pot. Stir, cover, and seal the pot. Pressure-cook on high for 20 minutes.

5 Do a quick pressure release, remove the bay leaves, and enjoy the chili while hot!

PER SERVING: *Calories 385; Fat 27g; Cholesterol 81mg; Sodium 681mg; Carbohydrate 15g (Dietary Fiber 5g, Sugar Alcohol 0g); Net Carbohydrate 10g; Protein 23g.*

Instant Pot Pot Roast

PREP TIME: 15 MIN	COOK TIME: 1 HR AND 20 MIN	YIELD: 8 SERVINGS

INGREDIENTS

3 pounds boneless beef chuck roast

1 teaspoon salt

1 teaspoon ground black pepper

2 teaspoons garlic powder

2 teaspoons Italian seasoning

1 tablespoon unsalted butter

½ cup chopped onions

1 cup sliced mushrooms

1 tablespoon tomato paste

1 tablespoon coconut aminos

2 cups beef broth

8 radishes, halved

1 cup cauliflower florets

1 cup chopped celery

1 cup broccoli florets

1 red bell pepper, sliced

2 sprigs rosemary

DIRECTIONS

1 Sprinkle the chuck roast with the salt and pepper, garlic powder, and Italian seasoning.

2 Turn the Instant Pot on to sauté and place the butter in the pot.

3 Add the seasoned chuck roast to the butter and sear on one side for 4 minutes; then flip and sear for another 4 minutes.

4 Add the onions and mushrooms and cook for 2 minutes.

5 Add the tomato paste, coconut aminos, and beef broth; then cover and seal the Instant pot. Cook on high pressure for 60 minutes.

6 Once the cooking time is up, do a quick pressure release.

7 Add the rest of the ingredients to the Instant Pot and seal again. Pressure-cook on high for 2 minutes.

8 Let the pressure release naturally. Then remove the meat from the pot and let it sit for 5 minutes before slicing. Discard the rosemary.

9 Divide the veggies and meat on plates and enjoy!

PER SERVING: *Calories 271; Fat 11g; Cholesterol 113mg; Sodium 420mg; Carbohydrate 6g (Dietary Fiber 2g, Sugar Alcohol 0g); Net Carbohydrate 4g; Protein 38g.*

Instant Pot Sausage and Peppers

PREP TIME: 10 MIN   **COOK TIME: 15 MIN**   **YIELD: 8 SERVINGS**

INGREDIENTS

¼ tablespoons olive oil

8 sweet Italian sausage links

1 large onion, sliced

4 garlic cloves, minced

2 cups chicken broth

4 red or green bell peppers, sliced

2 cups Rao's tomato sauce

DIRECTIONS

1 Place the olive oil into the Instant Pot and press sauté.

2 Add the sausage links and brown on each side for about 2 minutes.

3 Add the onions and garlic to the Instant Pot and sauté everything together for 5 minutes, stirring occasionally.

4 Add the chicken broth, bell peppers, and tomato sauce and stir.

5 Cover and seal the Instant Pot and cook on high pressure for 8 minutes.

6 Let the pressure release naturally; then open and enjoy!

7 Divide the sausage and peppers into meal-prep containers to have easy dinners or lunches for the week.

PER SERVING: Calories 523; Fat 46g; Cholesterol 87mg; Sodium 1,232mg; Carbohydrate 9g (Dietary Fiber 2g, Sugar Alcohol 0g); Net Carbohydrate 7g; Protein 18g.

Slow Cooker Stuffed Cabbage

PREP TIME: 20 MIN	COOK TIME: 4 HOURS	YIELD: 8 SERVINGS

INGREDIENTS

1 head cabbage

1½ pounds 90/10 ground beef

1 cup chopped onions

2 tablespoons minced garlic

2 large eggs

1 teaspoon salt

½ teaspoon ground black pepper

4 cups Rao's tomato sauce

DIRECTIONS

1 Cut the bottom ½ inch off the head of the cabbage and place the whole head in boiling water. Cook for about 2 to 3 minutes to soften the leaves.

2 Remove the cabbage from the water, let it cool until you can handle it easily and peel back the leaves from the head. Trim off the thick spine of the leaves to make them roll more easily. You want to get at least 12 to 16 large leaves.

3 In a large bowl, combine the ground beef, onions, garlic, eggs, salt and pepper. Mix well.

4 Scoop about ¼ cup of the ground beef mixture onto each cabbage leaf. Roll the cabbage leaf around the meat, folding the edges in as you roll, like you would a burrito.

5 Place the cabbage rolls in your slow cooker.

6 Pour the tomato sauce over the cabbage rolls and then cook on high for 4 hours.

PER SERVING: *Calories 352; Fat 25g; Cholesterol 100mg; Sodium 437mg; Carbohydrate 13g (Dietary Fiber 3g, Sugar Alcohol 0g); Net Carbohydrate 10g; Protein 19g.*

VARY IT! You can also cook the cabbage rolls in an Instant Pot. Follow the same directions but place the rolls in your Instant Pot, seal, and cook on high pressure for 10 minutes. Do a natural pressure release, and then enjoy!

Instant Pot Meatballs with Parmesan Sauce

| PREP TIME: 20 MIN | COOK TIME: 15 MIN | YIELD: 6 SERVINGS |

INGREDIENTS

Meatballs:

1½ pounds ground turkey

2 tablespoons chopped parsley

2 tablespoons chopped green onions

½ cup almond flour

½ cup grated Parmesan cheese

2 teaspoons minced garlic

2 large eggs

½ cup chicken broth

Parmesan Sauce:

½ cup unsalted butter

4 tablespoons minced garlic

8 ounces cream cheese (1 cup)

6 ounces grated Parmesan cheese

¼ cup fresh chopped basil

2 medium zucchinis, spiralized, for serving

DIRECTIONS

1 Place all the ingredients except the chicken broth for the turkey meatballs in a large bowl and mix well.

2 Scoop into meatballs into 2-tablespoon-sized balls, rolling them with your hands and setting them aside on a plate.

3 Add the chicken broth to the Instant Pot, and then add your Instant Pot trivet.

4 Stack the meatballs on the trivet. It's okay if they are piled on top of each other.

5 Cover and seal the Instant Pot and set the timer for high pressure for 7 minutes. Do a quick pressure release.

6 Open the Instant Pot and move the meatballs to a tray.

7 Make the Parmesan sauce. Place the butter in the Instant Pot and press sauté.

8 Add the garlic to the pot and sauté for 2 minutes.

9 Add the cream cheese, Parmesan cheese, and basil. Stir to melt the cheese sauce completely, making it nice and smooth.

10 Add the zoodles to the pot and toss in the sauce.

11 Divide the sauced zoodles among six bowls and then top each with the meatballs. Enjoy while hot.

PER SERVING: *Calories 683; Fat 54g; Cholesterol 245mg; Sodium 846mg; Carbohydrate 9g (Dietary Fiber 2g, Sugar Alcohol 0g); Net Carbohydrate 8g; Protein 43g.*

Chapter **22**

Meal Prep for the Week

We know the importance of planning, especially when you first begin on your keto journey. Having a fridge full of meals that you know are keto friendly can really help you stick to your diet goals. Meal prep can be for breakfast, lunch, or dinner. You can even prep your snacks for the week!

Look at the recipes in this chapter and pick the ones that catch your eye. Make a menu for the week, deciding which meal-prep recipes you'd like to make and which days you want to eat them. This can also help you decide how many portions you need to make.

Set aside one day when you can spend extra time in the kitchen, prepping your foods for the week. While it may take a bit of time that one day, you will be saving multiples of that time throughout the week. Keep this in mind as you prep your week's meals!

Meal prep can also help you stick to all your macro goals. While all the recipes in this book are keto-friendly, you may have specific macro targets you want to hit. Use your meal-prep days to calculate your macros and make sure the meals you are planning for each day fit into these goals. This makes your keto diet that much more successful.

TIP

If you plan on doing meal prep often, invest in some good glass containers. We like containers that are reusable and can stack in the fridge, keeping the meals you make neat and tidy. Buy containers that are sized for individual portions. You can exercise portion control, plan your macro intake, and ensure you are eating flavorful foods all through meal prep.

Keto Taco Pie

PREP TIME: 15 MIN | **COOK TIME: 35 MIN** | **YIELD: 8 SERVINGS**

INGREDIENTS

1 tablespoon olive oil

2 pounds 90/10 ground beef

1 cup salsa

4 tablespoons taco seasoning

1 tablespoon minced garlic

¾ cup heavy cream

4 large eggs

1 cup shredded cheddar cheese

1 cup shredded pepper jack cheese

DIRECTIONS

1 Preheat the oven to 350 degrees and spray a 9-x-13-inch casserole dish with cooking spray.

2 Heat a large skillet over medium-high heat and add the olive oil and ground beef. Cook the ground beef for only 5 minutes to break it up, but don't cook it fully. It will finish cooking in the oven later.

3 Drain most of the fat from the ground beef and add the salsa, taco seasoning, and garlic to the beef and stir.

4 Pour the ground beef mixture into the casserole dish and spread it into a flat layer.

5 Whisk together the heavy cream and eggs. Pour the mixture over the ground beef.

6 Sprinkle the top of the casserole dish with the cheeses.

7 Bake the taco pie for 30 minutes. The cheese will be melted, and the pie will be nice and firm.

8 Let the pie sit for at least 10 minutes before slicing and serving or storing in meal-prep containers.

PER SERVING: *Calories 546; Fat 44g; Cholesterol 218mg; Sodium 843mg; Carbohydrate 6g (Dietary Fiber 1g, Sugar Alcohol 0g); Net Carbohydrate 5g; Protein 30g.*

Kale and Chicken Caesar Salad

PREP TIME: 15 MIN	COOK TIME: 25 MIN	YIELD: 8 SERVINGS

INGREDIENTS

Homemade Dressing (see the following recipe)

4 boneless, skinless chicken thighs

2 tablespoons olive oil

1 teaspoon garlic powder

Salt and pepper

10 cups chopped kale

DIRECTIONS

1 Preheat the oven to 450 degrees.

2 Place the chicken thighs in a medium-sized baking dish. Drizzle with the olive oil; then sprinkle with the garlic powder and a little salt and pepper.

3 Bake the chicken for 25 minutes until the internal temperature is 150 degrees. Remove the dish from the oven and let the chicken cool for 10 minutes before chopping it into cubes.

4 Make the dressing (see the following recipe).

5 Place the chopped kale in a very large bowl and add the homemade dressing.

6 Divide among eight meal-prep containers and store in the fridge for four to six days. When ready to eat, add the chicken to the dressed kale and toss to coat.

Homemade Dressing

INGREDIENTS

4 cloves garlic

6 anchovies

2 teaspoons Dijon mustard

¾ cup olive oil

¼ cup fresh lemon juice

6 ounces grated Parmesan cheese

DIRECTIONS

Place all the ingredients in a food processor and blend until creamy and smooth.

PER SERVING: *Calories 454; Fat 35g; Cholesterol 112mg; Sodium 560mg; Carbohydrate 7g (Dietary Fiber 2g, Sugar Alcohol 0g); Net Carbohydrate 5g; Protein 31g.*

NOTE: Kale is hearty enough to not wilt in the fridge even with dressing on it, which is why this is such a great meal-prep salad.

Peri Peri Skillet Chicken

PREP TIME: 15 MIN	COOK TIME: 40 MIN	YIELD: 6 SERVINGS

INGREDIENTS

2 red bell peppers, chopped

4 tablespoons minced garlic

1 cup chopped white onions

¼ cup olive oil

1 tablespoon smoked paprika

1 tablespoon cayenne pepper

2 teaspoons salt

5 dried chilies

1 teaspoon ground black pepper

4 tablespoons fresh lemon juice

4 tablespoons apple cider vinegar

1 teaspoon dried rosemary

4 tablespoons unsalted butter

6 chicken thighs, cut into cubes

DIRECTIONS

1 Preheat the oven to 350 degrees.

2 Spread the bell peppers, garlic, and onions on a rimmed baking sheet.

3 Drizzle the vegetables with olive oil; then sprinkle with the paprika, cayenne, and salt.

4 Roast the vegetables in the oven for 20 minutes.

5 Remove the roasted veggies from the oven and place them in a blender. Add the dried chilies, ground black pepper, lemon juice, vinegar, and rosemary to the blender as well.

6 Puree the mixture until smooth and thick to finish making the Peri Peri sauce.

7 Place the butter in a very large skillet and melt over medium-high heat.

8 Add the chopped chicken and sauté for about 15 minutes, turning occasionally to brown all sides.

9 Pour the Peri Peri sauce into the pan and cook for another 2 minutes.

10 Divide the chicken and sauce among meal-prep containers to have pre-made meals all week!

PER SERVING: *Calories 437; Fat 25g; Cholesterol 202mg; Sodium 193mg; Carbohydrate 12g (Dietary Fiber 3g, Sugar Alcohol 0g); Net Carbohydrate 9g; Protein 40g.*

TIP: This recipe freezes quite well. Divide the finished recipe among meal-prep containers and freeze for up to 4 weeks. When ready to eat, allow a serving to thaw completely in the refrigerator, then reheat.

Creamy Parmesan Chicken with Spinach

PREP TIME: 10 MIN	COOK TIME: 20 MIN	YIELD: 8 SERVINGS

INGREDIENTS

2 tablespoons olive oil

8 boneless, skinless chicken thighs

½ cup unsalted butter

2 tablespoons minced garlic

1 cup chicken broth

1½ cups heavy cream

1 cup grated Parmesan cheese

1 teaspoon garlic powder

1 teaspoon salt

½ teaspoon ground black pepper

8 cups baby spinach, lightly packed

1 cup chopped sundried tomatoes

DIRECTIONS

1 In a very large skillet, heat the olive oil over medium-high heat. Sear the chicken on each side for 6 minutes. Remove the chicken from the pan and set it aside. Repeat if all the chicken doesn't fit in the pan.

2 Add the butter to the pan and let it melt.

3 Add the garlic and cook for 2 minutes, stirring occasionally.

4 Whisk the chicken broth into the pan, scraping the browned bits from the bottom.

5 Whisk in the heavy cream, Parmesan cheese, garlic powder, salt and pepper.

6 Add the spinach and stir to wilt.

7 Add the sundried tomatoes to the pan; then add the chicken back into the pan and cook for 2 more minutes.

8 Serve the creamy Parmesan chicken while hot or divide it into individual meal-prep containers.

PER SERVING: *Calories 605; Fat 42g; Cholesterol 282mg; Sodium 505mg; Carbohydrate 10g (Dietary Fiber 3g, Sugar Alcohol 0g); Net Carbohydrate 7g; Protein 46g.*

TIP: This recipe freezes quite well. Divide the finished recipe among meal-prep containers and freeze for up to 4 weeks. When ready to eat, allow a serving to thaw completely in the refrigerator, then reheat.

Chicken Enchilada Casserole

PREP TIME: 5 MIN	COOK TIME: 20 MIN	YIELD: 6 SERVINGS

INGREDIENTS

1 tablespoon olive oil

½ cup chopped onions

1 teaspoon salt

½ teaspoon ground black pepper

1 tablespoon minced garlic

3 tablespoons chili powder

2 cups Rao's tomato sauce

6 chicken thighs, cooked and shredded

1 (4-ounce) can diced mild chili peppers

½ cup minced cilantro

2 cups shredded cheddar cheese, divided

½ cup sour cream, for serving

DIRECTIONS

1 Preheat the oven to 400 degrees and grease a 7-x-11-inch casserole dish.

2 Place the olive oil in a large skillet and heat over medium-high.

3 Add the onions, salt and pepper and cook for 5 minutes to soften the onions.

4 Add the garlic, chili powder, tomato sauce, and a ½ cup of water and stir. Bring the sauce to a simmer and cook for 5 minutes to thicken to the consistency of enchilada sauce. Set aside.

5 In a large bowl, combine the chicken, enchilada sauce, chili peppers, cilantro, and 1 cup of cheese.

6 Spread the chicken mixture in the prepared casserole dish, then sprinkle with the remaining cup of cheese.

7 Bake for 10 minutes until the cheese is melted and the mixture is bubbling.

8 Divide the recipe into individual meal-prep containers. When ready to eat, drizzle with sour cream and serve!

PER SERVING: *Calories 524; Fat 32g; Cholesterol 230mg; Sodium 782mg; Carbohydrate 9g (Dietary Fiber 2g, Sugar Alcohol 0g); Net Carbohydrate 7g; Protein 49g.*

TIP: You can use a spatula to cut the casserole into six equal pieces and place them in meal-prep containers. Store them in the fridge for up to a week and reheat anytime you need a quick, keto meal.

Tuna Salad Lettuce Wraps

PREP TIME: 15 MIN	COOK TIME: NONE	YIELD: 6 SERVINGS

INGREDIENTS

3 (5½ ounce) cans tuna in water

3 large hard-boiled eggs, chopped

6 tablespoons mayonnaise

2 tablespoons Dijon mustard

1 cup chopped celery

2 teaspoons Sriracha

1 teaspoon garlic powder

½ teaspoon salt

½ teaspoon ground black pepper

1 teaspoon fresh lemon juice

½ cup chopped parsley

6 large romaine lettuce leaves

DIRECTIONS

1 To make the tuna salad, place all the ingredients except the lettuce leaves in a large bowl.

2 Mash together, mixing everything well. Store the tuna salad in an airtight container.

3 When ready to eat, place the lettuce leaves on a flat work surface and add ¾ cup of tuna salad to the center of each leaf.

4 Roll up each leaf around the tuna salad, like a burrito, so the salad is completely enclosed.

PER SERVING: *Calories 278; Fat 15g; Cholesterol 142mg; Sodium 617mg; Carbohydrate 2g (Dietary Fiber 1g, Sugar Alcohol 0g); Net Carbohydrate 1g; Protein 34g.*

Keto Buddha Bowl

PREP TIME: 15 MIN	COOK TIME: 20 MIN	YIELD: 6 SERVINGS

INGREDIENTS

¾ cup olive oil, divided

1 red bell pepper

1 orange bell pepper

1 yellow bell pepper

1 red onion, sliced

1 carrot, thinly sliced into matchsticks

1 tablespoon minced garlic

6 boneless, skinless chicken breasts, cut in half lengthwise

Salt and pepper

1 cup plain Greek yogurt

¼ cup fresh lemon juice

¼ cup low carb pancake syrup

DIRECTIONS

1 Add 2 tablespoons of the olive oil to a large skillet and heat over medium–high heat.

2 Slice all the peppers and add to the skillet along with the onions, carrot sticks, and garlic. Sauté for 10 minutes, stirring occasionally. The peppers should be soft and browned.

3 Remove the veggies from the pan and place them into six meal-prep containers.

4 Add 2 more tablespoons of the olive oil to the skillet, and then add the chicken breasts. Season with a little salt and pepper. Then sear the chicken for 5 minutes on each side, making it golden brown and crisp.

5 Place one chicken breast in each meal-prep container along with the roasted veggies.

6 Place the yogurt, lemon juice, pancake syrup, a little salt and pepper, and the remaining olive oil in a small bowl and whisk together. Store the dressing in a separate container.

PER SERVING: *Calories 625; Fat 45g; Cholesterol 118mg; Sodium 143mg; Carbohydrate 15g (Dietary Fiber 5g, Sugar Alcohol 2g); Net Carbohydrate 8g; Protein 41g.*

TIP: Whenever you're eating the Buddha bowls, pour some of the dressing over the meal.

Feta and Pepper Egg Cups

PREP TIME: 10 MIN	COOK TIME: 25 MIN	YIELD: 6 SERVINGS (2 EGG CUPS PER SERVING)

INGREDIENTS

2 tablespoons olive oil

1 cup red bell pepper, chopped

2 teaspoons minced garlic

2 cups baby spinach, lightly packed

8 large eggs

¼ cup heavy cream

1 teaspoon salt

½ teaspoon black pepper

1 cup feta cheese

DIRECTIONS

1 Preheat the oven to 400 degrees and grease the 12 wells of a muffin pan.

2 Pour the olive oil in a large skillet and heat over medium-high heat.

3 Add the chopped peppers and garlic to the skillet and cook for 5 minutes.

4 Add the spinach to the pan and stir until it is wilted. Remove the pan from the heat.

5 In a medium bowl, whisk the eggs and heavy cream together.

6 Add the salt and pepper, and feta to the egg mixture.

7 Scoop the cooked veggies into the prepared muffin cups, dividing the veggies evenly.

8 Pour the egg and cheese mixture into each muffin cup, on top of the veggies.

9 Bake the egg cups in the oven for 16 minutes. The eggs should be completely set.

10 Enjoy warm or cold. Store in the fridge for up to a week in an airtight container.

PER SERVING: *Calories 233; Fat 19g; Cholesterol 249mg; Sodium 324mg; Carbohydrate 4g (Dietary Fiber 1g, Sugar Alcohol 0g); Net Carbohydrate 4g; Protein 12g.*

TIP: These egg cups make easy, grab-and-go breakfasts!

Salmon Kale Salad

PREP TIME: 15 MIN | COOK TIME: 15 MIN | YIELD: 6 SERVINGS

INGREDIENTS

6 (4-ounce) salmon filets

Salt and pepper

2 tablespoons fresh chopped rosemary

1 medium lemon, sliced

6 cups kale, sliced

6 tablespoons grated Parmesan cheese

6 tablespoons lemon juice

1 teaspoon lemon zest

3 tablespoons olive oil

6 tablespoons sunflower seeds

3 tablespoons pistachios

1 cup halved cherry tomatoes, for serving

DIRECTIONS

1 Preheat the oven to 400 degrees. Line a rimmed baking sheet with aluminum foil.

2 Place the salmon on the prepared baking sheet and season with a little salt and pepper and the rosemary.

3 Place the lemon slices on top of the salmon and bake for 15 minutes. The internal temperature of the salmon should be 145 degrees. Set aside to cool.

4 Combine all the remaining ingredients except the cherry tomatoes in a large bowl and toss them together well.

5 Divide the salad among six meal-prep containers and top each one with a salmon filet. Top with the cherry tomatoes. Store in the fridge in airtight containers.

PER SERVING: *Calories 448; Fat 31g; Cholesterol 67mg; Sodium 185mg; Carbohydrate 12g (Dietary Fiber 4g, Sugar Alcohol 0g); Net Carbohydrate 8g; Protein 32g.*

TIP: This makes an easy lunch or dinner option. If desired, you can quickly reheat the salmon in the microwave for 1 minute to heat it back up.

NOTE: Kale is hearty enough to not wilt in the fridge even with dressing on it, which is why this is such a great meal-prep salad.

5
Enjoying Keto Drinks, Snacks, and Desserts

IN THIS PART . . .

Try a variety of different keto drinks and smoothies.

Get your munch on with keto snacks.

Keep your sweet tooth happy with mouth-watering desserts.

Chapter **23**

Drinks

D rinks are a huge source of hidden carbs. Sodas, juices, and most alcoholic mixed drinks are full of sugars that you may have never noticed until you started following a keto diet. All these carb-loaded drinks need to be eliminated right away. But then, what's left to drink?

There are lots of delicious, keto-friendly drinks that you can enjoy. From low-carb, high-fat smoothies to energy drinks to interesting teas and coffees, you will never grow tired of keto drinks. Water is always a great option as well and a safe choice if you are ever wary of a drink menu while dining out. You can never go wrong with water.

Keto drinks are often sweetened with low-carb sweeteners like erythritol, Splenda, or even bacon syrup. These sweeteners help make drinks taste good while keeping to your dietary restrictions. You can find lots of canned drinks that are low carb, and even some of your favorite sodas may come in low-carb form.

Zero-carb drinks are a great way to give yourself a little treat between meals. A tasty drink can help you stay full until your next meal and satisfy any cravings you may have for sweetness. Keep in mind that unsweetened drinks with no added sweeteners whatsoever are also quite refreshing. Try plain, black tea or some simple infused water. You will be surprised by how the most basic drinks sometimes turn out to be the best!

Staying low-carb while drinking alcohol can be a bit more difficult because you don't get nutrition labels when you order a drink at a bar or restaurant. Here's a quick guide on the types of alcohol you can safely consume.

Clear liquors at about 40 percent alcohol are a safe bet and are considered keto at zero total carbs! Acceptable clear liquors include:

» Vodka

» Tequila

» Gin

» Whiskey

» Rum

» Scotch

» Brandy

» Cognac

Following are the carb contents for wines and beers that are okay to have a few servings of on a keto diet.

Red wines (5-ounce serving):

» **Cabernet Sauvignon:** 120 calories, 3.8 carbs

» **Pinot Noir:** 121 calories, 3.4 carbs

» **Merlot:** 120 calories, 3.7 carbs

White wines (5-ounce serving):

» **Pinot Grigio:** 122 calories, 3.2 carbs

» **Sauvignon Blanc:** 122 calories, 2.7 carbs

» **Chardonnay:** 118 calories, 3.7 carbs

» **Riesling:** 118 calories, 5.5 carbs

» **Champagne:** 96 calories, 1.5 carbs

Light beers (12-ounce serving):

>> **Bud Select 55:** 55 calories, 1.9 carbs

>> **MGD 64:** 64 calories, 2.4 carbs

>> **Rolling Rock Green Light:** 92 calories, 2.4 carbs

>> **Michelob Ultra:** 95 calories, 2.6 carbs

>> **Bud Select:** 99 calories, 3.1 carbs

>> **Miller Lite:** 96 calories, 3.2 carbs

>> **Natural Light:** 95 calories, 3.2 carbs

>> **Michelob Ultra Amber:** 114 calories, 3.7 carbs

>> **Coors Light:** 102 calories, 5 carbs

>> **Amstel Light:** 95 calories, 5 carbs

>> **Bud Light:** 110 calories, 6.6 carbs

When drinking mixed drinks, try to stick to drinks that either omit sweeteners like simple syrup, or ask the bartender to skip the sugary mixers. Here are some of the more common ones you will want to avoid:

>> Blue curaçao

>> Frozen margarita mixes

>> Grenadine

>> Simple syrup

>> Sugary syrups

>> Triple sec

>> Whiskey sour mix

Avocado Smoothie

PREP TIME: 5 MIN	COOK TIME: NONE	YIELD: 2 SERVINGS

INGREDIENTS

1 cup unsweetened almond milk

2 tablespoons powdered erythritol

2 cups ice

1 large avocado

DIRECTIONS

1　Place all the ingredients into a blender and puree until smooth.

2　Pour into two glasses and enjoy.

PER SERVING: *Calories 179; Fat 16g; Cholesterol 0mg; Sodium 102mg; Carbohydrate 21g (Dietary Fiber 8g, Sugar Alcohol 12g); Net Carbohydrate 2g; Protein 3g.*

Raspberry Mint Smoothie

INGREDIENTS

1 large avocado, peeled and pitted

1 cup frozen raspberries

1 tablespoon lemon juice

4 fresh mint leaves

1½ cups unsweetened canned coconut milk

1 tablespoon powdered erythritol

DIRECTIONS

1 Place all the ingredients into a blender and puree until very smooth.

2 Pour into two glasses and enjoy.

PER SERVING: *Calories 228; Fat 19g; Cholesterol 0mg; Sodium 16mg; Carbohydrate 23g (Dietary Fiber 11g, Sugar Alcohol 6g); Net Carbohydrate 6g; Protein 3g.*

Keto Dalgona Coffee

PREP TIME: 5 MIN	COOK TIME: 1 MIN	YIELD: 1 SERVING

INGREDIENTS

2 tablespoons instant coffee powder

2 tablespoons granular erythritol

2 tablespoons boiling water

1 cup unsweetened canned coconut milk

2 tablespoons heavy cream

DIRECTIONS

1 Place the instant coffee, erythritol, and boiling water in a small bowl.

2 Use an electric hand mixer, whisk, or milk frother to whip the mix until thick and frothy.

3 Place the coconut milk and heavy cream in a mug and heat in the microwave on high for 45 seconds.

4 Scoop the foamy coffee mix over the warm milk; then enjoy!

PER SERVING: *Calories 170; Fat 16g; Cholesterol 41mg; Sodium 25mg; Carbohydrate 30g (Dietary Fiber 0g, Sugar Alcohol 24g); Net Carbohydrate 6g; Protein 2g.*

Cucumber Limeade

INGREDIENTS

2 medium cucumbers

2 tablespoons low-carb pancake syrup

½ cup water

1 teaspoon salt

¼ cup lime juice

Ice

½ cup sparkling water

DIRECTIONS

1 Peel one cucumber and then place it in a blender along with the pancake syrup, water, salt, and lime juice. Blend until smooth.

2 Pour the mixture through a fine-mesh strainer.

3 Use a peeler to peel long strips of the other cucumber. Place two cucumber strips in two tall glasses, letting the thin cucumber slices spiral in the glass.

4 Fill the cucumber-lined glasses with ice.

5 Pour the cucumber limeade into each glass, and top each with sparkling water.

6 Stir once or twice with a straw and then enjoy while the drinks are cold and fresh.

PER SERVING: *Calories 44; Fat 0g; Cholesterol 0mg; Sodium 7mg; Carbohydrate 14g (Dietary Fiber 6g, Sugar Alcohol 3g); Net Carbohydrate 6g; Protein 1g.*

Cranberry Smoothie

INGREDIENTS

2 cups ice

¼ cup cranberries

½ cup almonds

2 tablespoons low-carb pancake syrup

2 tablespoons powdered erythritol

1 cup plain Greek yogurt

DIRECTIONS

1 Place all the ingredients into a blender and puree until smooth.

2 Pour into two glasses and enjoy.

PER SERVING: *Calories 356; Fat 25g; Cholesterol 19mg; Sodium 78mg; Carbohydrate 23g (Dietary Fiber 10g, Sugar Alcohol 3g); Net Carbohydrate 10g; Protein 18g.*

Coconut Almond Smoothie

PREP TIME: 5 MIN	COOK TIME: NONE	YIELD: 1 SERVING

INGREDIENTS

½ cup canned coconut milk

½ cup unsweetened coconut milk (refrigerated)

2 tablespoons almond butter

1 tablespoon shredded, unsweetened coconut

½ cup ice

1 tablespoon hemp seeds

DIRECTIONS

1 Place all the ingredients into a blender and puree until very smooth.

2 Pour into a glass and enjoy.

PER SERVING: *Calories 754; Fat 74g; Cholesterol 0mg; Sodium 44mg; Carbohydrate 18g (Dietary Fiber 8g, Sugar Alcohol 0g); Net Carbohydrate 9g; Protein 15g.*

Coconut Coffee Smoothie

INGREDIENTS

1 cup unsweetened canned coconut milk

½ cup canned coconut milk

½ cup cold brew coffee

1 tablespoon almond butter

1 tablespoon unsweetened shredded coconut

1 cup ice

DIRECTIONS

1 Place all the ingredients into a blender and puree until smooth.

2 Pour into two glasses and enjoy.

PER SERVING: *Calories 201; Fat 21g; Cholesterol 0mg; Sodium 13mg; Carbohydrate 4g (Dietary Fiber 1g, Sugar Alcohol 0g); Net Carbohydrate 3g; Protein 3g.*

Green Tea Smoothie

INGREDIENTS

1 cup unsweetened canned coconut milk

2 teaspoons matcha green tea powder

2 cups baby spinach, lightly packed

1 cup frozen coconut chunks

1 tablespoon granular erythritol

1 cup ice

DIRECTIONS

1 Place all the ingredients into a blender and puree until very smooth.

2 Pour into two glasses and serve with keto whipped cream if desired. Enjoy while frozen.

PER SERVING: *Calories 230; Fat 21g; Cholesterol 0mg; Sodium 46mg; Carbohydrate 16g (Dietary Fiber 6g, Sugar Alcohol 6g); Net Carbohydrate 5g; Protein 3g.*

Chapter **24**

Snacks

Snacks can be important to the success of any diet. If you don't allow yourself to indulge in a snack every now and then, you are far more likely to quit your diet. Your body may be craving a quick bite or a salty snack to get a little extra energy, and you should listen to what it wants. You will be happier and healthier when you incorporate some keto snacks into your daily routine.

We think that snacks should be easy to make. They are not an elaborate, main course but something small and fast. All our recipes are simple to put together but still give you lots of great flavor and feed your need for a snacky type of food.

Just as you plan your main keto meals, try to also plan out your snacks for the day or even for the week. Use these snacks to boost your macros in the areas you may need. Add some extra fats by making energy balls or get a little bit more protein with some easy cheese chips. Meal-prep your snacks for the week so they are ready for you to grab and go. Snacks are meant to be convenient, and these recipes help you stay on the keto track while also smiling all day long.

Pork Rind Nachos

PREP TIME: 10 MIN | COOK TIME: 4 MIN | YIELD: 2 SERVINGS

INGREDIENTS

2 ounces pork rinds

1 ounce sliced pickled jalapeños

¼ cup chopped red onions

½ cup chopped tomatoes

1 cup shredded cheddar cheese

¼ cup sour cream, for serving (optional)

¼ cup guacamole, for serving (optional)

DIRECTIONS

1 Set the oven to broil and line a rimmed baking sheet with aluminum foil.

2 Spread the pork rinds across the lined baking sheet. Sprinkle the jalapeño, onions, tomatoes, and cheese over the top.

3 Broil for about 3 to 4 minutes to melt the cheese completely.

4 Enjoy with a side of sour cream and guacamole, if desired.

PER SERVING: *Calories 444; Fat 34g; Cholesterol 108mg; Sodium 827mg; Carbohydrate 5g (Dietary Fiber 1g, Sugar Alcohol 0g); Net Carbohydrate 4g; Protein 29g.*

Cucumber and Shrimp Rollups

PREP TIME: 15 MIN	COOK TIME: NONE	YIELD: 4 SERVINGS

INGREDIENTS

2 English cucumbers, sliced thinly lengthwise into long, wide strips

4 ounces cream cheese (½ cup), softened

2 teaspoons chopped chives

1 clove garlic, minced

¼ teaspoon salt

¼ teaspoon ground black pepper

½ pound large shrimp, peeled, deveined, cooked

DIRECTIONS

1 Lay the cucumber slices on a piece of paper towel and pat dry. (You should have the same number of cucumber slices as pieces of shrimp.)

2 In a large bowl, mix the cream cheese, chives, garlic, salt and pepper.

3 Spread about 1 tablespoon of the cream cheese mixture across each cucumber slice.

4 Roll up the cucumbers into tight pinwheels.

5 Skewer a cooked shrimp with a toothpick and then pierce the toothpick through the cucumber roll to secure closed.

6 Chill the cucumber rolls until ready to enjoy.

PER SERVING: *Calories 151; Fat 11g; Cholesterol 103mg; Sodium 427mg; Carbohydrate 4g (Dietary Fiber 1g, Sugar Alcohol 0g); Net Carbohydrate 3g; Protein 10g.*

NOTE: We prefer English cucumbers because they contain fewer seeds and are less fragile.

Cayenne Kale Chips

| PREP TIME: 15 MIN | COOK TIME: 15 MIN | YIELD: 4 SERVINGS |

INGREDIENTS

4 cups chopped kale, stems removed

1 teaspoon sea salt

1 tablespoon olive oil

1½ teaspoons powdered cayenne pepper

1 tablespoon soy sauce

DIRECTIONS

1 Preheat the oven to 300 degrees.

2 Place the kale in a large bowl and toss it with all the other ingredients.

3 Spread the seasoned kale on a rimmed baking sheet in a flat layer.

4 Bake the chips in the oven for 15 minutes or until crispy. The edges of the kale should be slightly browned.

5 Let the chips cool a few minutes. Enjoy immediately.

PER SERVING: *Calories 41; Fat 4g; Cholesterol 0mg; Sodium 807mg; Carbohydrate 2g (Dietary Fiber 1g, Sugar Alcohol 0g); Net Carbohydrate 1g; Protein 1g.*

Sweet Coconut Balls

PREP TIME: 10 MIN	COOK TIME: NONE	YIELD: 5 SERVINGS (4 BALLS EACH)

INGREDIENTS

1 cup almond flour

3½ cups unsweetened shredded coconut, divided

½ cup low-carb pancake syrup

2 tablespoons granular

⅓ cup canned coconut milk

DIRECTIONS

1 Place the almond flour, 3 cups of the shredded coconut, pancake syrup, erythritol, and coconut milk into a food processor and puree until a thick dough forms.

2 Scoop the mixture into 2-tablespoon-sized balls and roll the balls with your hands to make about 20 balls.

3 Use the food processor to pulse the remaining shredded coconut, making finer pieces, and pour into a small bowl.

4 Roll the balls in the finely shredded coconut and then store in an airtight container in the fridge.

PER SERVING: *Calories 573; Fat 53g; Cholesterol 0mg; Sodium 24mg; Carbohydrate 36g (Dietary Fiber 19g, Sugar Alcohol 9g); Net Carbohydrate 8g; Protein 9g.*

Jalapeño Cheese Crisps

PREP TIME: 5 MIN   COOK TIME: 10 MIN   YIELD: 4 SERVINGS

INGREDIENTS

¾ cup shredded cheddar cheese

¾ cup shredded jalapeño pepper Jack cheese

Salt and pepper to taste

1 fresh jalapeño

DIRECTIONS

1 Preheat the oven to 400 degrees. Lightly grease the wells of a 12-cup muffin pan. (You can use multiple tins to make all the chips at once.)

2 Mix the two cheeses together in a large bowl. Add salt and pepper.

3 Scoop about 2 tablespoons of the shredded cheese mixture into each muffin cup.

4 Cut the top stem area off the jalapeño. Use the point of a knife to cut the seeds out of the center of the jalapeño, keeping the jalapeño whole. Discard the seeds.

5 Slice the jalapeño into twelve rings.

6 Place one jalapeño ring in the center of each cheese cup.

7 Bake for 8 to 10 minutes, until the cheese has melted and is bubbling. The edges of the cheese should just be turning golden brown. The jalapeño rings should also be starting to brown.

8 Let the cheese chips cool in the pan until hardened.

9 Remove the chips from the muffin pan and enjoy fresh or store refrigerated in an airtight container.

PER SERVING: *Calories 140; Fat 11g; Cholesterol 34mg; Sodium 221mg; Carbohydrate 1g (Dietary Fiber 0g, Sugar Alcohol 0g); Net Carbohydrate 1g; Protein 9g.*

Peanut Butter Mocha Energy Balls

PREP TIME: 10 MIN	COOK TIME: NONE	YIELD: 8 SERVINGS (2 BALLS EACH)

INGREDIENTS

⅓ cup low-carb pancake syrup

2 teaspoons instant coffee powder

1 cup unsweetened peanut butter

2 tablespoons powdered erythritol

⅓ cup coconut flour

⅓ cup almond flour

¼ cup unsweetened cocoa powder

DIRECTIONS

1 Add the syrup to a medium-sized microwave-safe bowl. Microwave on high for 30 seconds.

2 Add the instant coffee powder to the syrup and stir until it dissolves.

3 Stir in the rest of the ingredients together to make a thick, smooth dough.

4 Scoop the dough into 2-tablespoon-sized balls. Roll the balls with your hands so they are smooth.

5 Toss the energy balls in a little extra cocoa powder or leave plain.

6 Store in an airtight container in the fridge.

PER SERVING: *Calories 255; Fat 20g; Cholesterol 0mg; Sodium 16mg; Carbohydrate 17g (Dietary Fiber 8g, Sugar Alcohol 2g); Net Carbohydrate 8g; Protein 9g.*

Greek Yogurt Dip with Cucumber Sticks

PREP TIME: 5 MIN	COOK TIME: NONE	YIELD: 4 SERVINGS

INGREDIENTS

3 medium cucumbers

1 cup plain Greek yogurt

1 tablespoon lemon juice

2 teaspoons fresh chopped dill

1 teaspoon minced garlic

¼ teaspoon salt

¼ teaspoon ground black pepper

DIRECTIONS

1 Quarter two cucumbers lengthwise and set aside on a serving tray or platter. Grate the remaining cucumber.

2 Stir all the ingredients except the quartered cucumbers together in a medium bowl. Chill the dip in the fridge for at least an hour.

3 Serve the chilled dip with the quartered cucumbers.

PER SERVING: *Calories 83; Fat 4g; Cholesterol 10mg; Sodium 37mg; Carbohydrate 6g (Dietary Fiber 1g, Sugar Alcohol 0g); Net Carbohydrate 5g; Protein 6g.*

TIP: You can also use your favorite keto chips or veggies in place of the cucumbers for dipping.

Blueberry Crème Fraîche Bowls

INGREDIENTS

1 cup crème fraîche

¼ cup powdered erythritol

1 teaspoon lemon zest

3 tablespoons lemon juice

2 cups blueberries

DIRECTIONS

1. Place the crème fraîche, erythritol, lemon zest, and lemon juice in a bowl and mix.

2. Divide the crème fraîche among four bowls.

3. Top each bowl with ½ cup blueberries.

4. Enjoy cold.

PER SERVING: *Calories 152; Fat 11g; Cholesterol 29mg; Sodium 27mg; Carbohydrate 25g (Dietary Fiber 2g, Sugar Alcohol 12g); Net Carbohydrate 11g; Protein 2g.*

Chapter **25**

Desserts

The cravings for sweet foods can be pretty intense when you are first starting a keto diet. It changes your view of desserts and can be a hard adjustment. Your body craves sugar you aren't supposed to have (because we want what we can't have!).

The good news is there's nothing to worry about! There are so many desserts that you *can* have. You need to know what to make and the ingredients to use. Natural sweeteners like erythritol, monk fruit, and stevia help you create keto-friendly desserts that satisfy your need for sweets while sticking to your keto diet.

Unchecked cravings have been shown to be very harmful to diets. While self-control is important, you must also satisfy your food cravings. Otherwise, you get stuck focusing on what you *can't* have rather than enjoying what you *can* have while on your diet. With the help of some keto sweeteners and a few low-carb ingredient replacements, you can satisfy your cravings and enjoy the foods you want but in a low-carb way.

In this chapter, you find tons of desserts that you may have thought were off-limits on the keto diet. You'll be amazed by how delicious keto desserts can be. The best part is that they are healthy, within your daily macros, and not difficult to put together. So, if you have a few minutes, try one of these keto dessert recipes.

Keto Strawberry Cake

INGREDIENTS

Whipped cream (see the following recipe)

2 large eggs

¼ cup butter, softened

1 cup strawberries, pureed

1 cup granular erythritol

⅛ teaspoon salt

1 teaspoon vanilla extract

1⅓ cups almond flour

4 tablespoons coconut flour

2 teaspoons baking powder

DIRECTIONS

1 Preheat the oven to 350 degrees and grease a 9-inch-square baking pan.

2 Mix the eggs, butter, strawberry puree, erythritol, salt, and vanilla in a large bowl, whisking until smooth.

3 Add the almond flour, coconut flour, and baking powder and stir again until smooth.

4 Pour the batter into the prepared pan and spread evenly.

5 Bake for 15 to 20 minutes. The center of the cake should be set and spring back to the touch. Let the cake cool completely.

6 Make the whipped cream (see the following recipe). Pipe or scoop the whipped cream on top of the cake and enjoy immediately.

Whipped Cream

INGREDIENTS

1 cup heavy cream

¼ cup powdered erythritol

½ teaspoon cream of tartar

DIRECTIONS

1 Place the heavy cream and erythritol in a medium-sized bowl and whisk until stiff peaks form.

2 Whisk in the cream of tartar.

PER SERVING: *Calories 268; Fat 25g; Cholesterol 85mg; Sodium 144mg; Carbohydrate 34g (Dietary Fiber 3g, Sugar Alcohol 27g); Net Carbohydrate 4g; Protein 6g.*

Keto Blondies

PREP TIME: 10 MIN   COOK TIME: 21 MIN   YIELD: 16 SERVINGS

INGREDIENTS

1⅓ cups almond flour

1 teaspoon baking powder

½ teaspoon salt

½ cup butter

1 cup brown sugar erythritol

1 large egg

1 teaspoon vanilla extract

DIRECTIONS

1   Preheat the oven to 350 degrees and grease a 9-inch-square baking pan.

2   Whisk the almond flour, baking powder, and salt together in a large bowl. Set aside.

3   Place the butter in a microwave-safe bowl and melt in the microwave on high for 45 seconds.

4   Whisk the erythritol into the melted butter.

5   Whisk the egg and vanilla into the butter and sweetener mixture.

6   Add the wet ingredients to the dry ingredient bowl and stir until smooth.

7   Pour the batter into the prepared pan.

8   Bake for 20 minutes.

9   Let the blondies cool for 15 minutes before slicing and serving.

PER SERVING: *Calories 110; Fat 11g; Cholesterol 25mg; Sodium 100mg; Carbohydrate 14g (Dietary Fiber 1g, Sugar Alcohol 12g); Net Carbohydrate 1g; Protein 3g.*

No-Bake Peanut Butter Bars

PREP TIME: 10 MIN	COOK TIME: 2 MIN	YIELD: 8 SERVINGS

INGREDIENTS

1 cup almond flour

4 tablespoons unsalted butter

¼ cup powdered erythritol

⅔ cup creamy peanut butter

1 teaspoon vanilla extract

¾ cup Lily's dark chocolate chips

DIRECTIONS

1 Line an 8-inch-square pan with parchment paper.

2 Place the almond flour, butter, erythritol, peanut butter, and vanilla in a medium-sized bowl and mix well.

3 Scoop the batter into the parchment-lined pan and spread evenly.

4 Place the chocolate chips in a small microwave-safe bowl. Microwave on high, heating and stirring in 30-second increments until the chocolate is melted.

5 Pour the melted chocolate over the batter and spread across the top evenly.

6 Refrigerate for 2 hours until the layers are firm. Then slice into bars and enjoy!

PER SERVING: *Calories 343; Fat 32g; Cholesterol 23mg; Sodium 5mg; Carbohydrate 24g (Dietary Fiber 7g, Sugar Alcohol 9g); Net Carbohydrate 7g; Protein 9g.*

Cinnamon Sugar Donut Bites

PREP TIME: 15 MIN	COOK TIME: 8 MIN	YIELD: 6 SERVINGS (2 BITES EACH)

INGREDIENTS

Donut Batter:

¼ cup melted unsalted butter

1 cup almond flour

2 tablespoons coconut flour

1¼ teaspoons baking powder

1 teaspoon ground cinnamon

¼ cup granular erythritol

½ teaspoon salt

2 tablespoons sour cream

Coating:

2 teaspoons cinnamon

⅓ cup powdered erythritol

¼ cup unsalted butter, melted

DIRECTIONS

1 Preheat the oven to 325 degrees and line a baking sheet with parchment paper.

2 Place all the donut batter ingredients in a medium-sized bowl and stir to mix into a thick dough. If it is too thick to stir, add 2 tablespoons of hot water.

3 Scoop the dough into 1-inch balls and roll them between your hands. Place each ball on the parchment-lined baking sheet, spacing them about 2 inches apart.

4 Bake for 8 minutes.

5 Let the doughnut bites cool enough to touch them.

6 Make the coating: Place the cinnamon and powdered erythritol in a small bowl and stir together.

7 Dip each doughnut bite in the melted butter and then roll it in the cinnamon mixture. Enjoy while warm!

PER SERVING: *Calories 266; Fat 26g; Cholesterol 43mg; Sodium 279mg; Carbohydrate 25g (Dietary Fiber 4g, Sugar Alcohol 19g); Net Carbohydrate 3g; Protein 5g.*

Dark Chocolate Brownies

PREP TIME: 10 MIN	COOK TIME: 19 MIN	YIELD: 8 SERVINGS

INGREDIENTS

½ cup almond flour

2 tablespoons coconut flour

¼ cup unsweetened cocoa powder

¾ cup granular erythritol

½ teaspoon baking powder

½ cup unsalted butter

½ cup Lily's dark chocolate chips

1 teaspoon vanilla extract

3 large eggs

DIRECTIONS

1 Preheat the oven to 350 degrees and line an 8-inch-square pan with parchment paper.

2 In a large bowl, whisk together the almond flour, coconut flour, cocoa powder, erythritol, and baking powder.

3 Heat the butter in a microwave on high for 30 seconds in a medium-sized, microwave-safe bowl. Add the chocolate chips and whisk to melt the chips in the butter. Allow to cool for a minute to avoid cooking the eggs in the next step.

4 Whisk the vanilla and eggs into the melted chocolate mix, and then pour the chocolate into the dry ingredients. Whisk everything together until smooth but stir slowly, so the brownies don't become too aerated and cakey when baked.

5 Pour the batter into the parchment-lined pan and bake for 18 minutes.

6 Let cool for at least 15 minutes before slicing and serving.

PER SERVING: *Calories 217; Fat 20g; Cholesterol 121mg; Sodium 52mg; Carbohydrate 29g (Dietary Fiber 5g, Sugar Alcohol 20g); Net Carbohydrate 3g; Protein 5g.*

Raspberry Almond Cake

PREP TIME: 10 MIN	COOK TIME: 35 MIN	YIELD: 8 SERVINGS

INGREDIENTS

Cake Batter:

2 cups almond flour

¼ cup coconut flour

1 tablespoon baking powder

¼ teaspoon salt

½ cup unsalted butter

1 cup granulated erythritol

3 large eggs

1 teaspoon almond extract

½ cup almond milk

Filling:

8 ounces cream cheese (1 cup)

½ cup powdered erythritol

1 large egg

1 teaspoon almond extract

1½ cups raspberries

¼ cup sliced almonds

DIRECTIONS

1 Preheat the oven to 325 degrees and grease a 9-inch spring-form pan with butter.

2 Place the almond flour, coconut flour, baking powder, and salt in a medium-sized bowl.

3 In a large bowl, beat the butter and erythritol until fluffy. Add the eggs and almond extract and mix together.

4 Add the dry ingredients to the butter mixture and blend into a smooth batter.

5 Add the almond milk and mix well.

6 Make the filling: In a separate large bowl, beat the cream cheese and powdered erythritol together until fluffy.

7 Add the egg and almond extract and mix again.

8 Fold in the raspberries and almonds.

9 Pour two-thirds of the cake batter into the pan, then add the raspberry filling, scooping spoonfuls around the pan evenly.

10 Pour the remaining cake batter over the raspberry filling and then bake for 35 minutes.

11 Let the cake cool for at least an hour before slicing and serving.

PER SERVING: *Calories 447; Fat 40g; Cholesterol 142mg; Sodium 363mg; Carbohydrate 49g (Dietary Fiber 6g, Sugar Alcohol 36g); Net Carbohydrate 7g; Protein 12g.*

Strawberry Walnut Yogurt

INGREDIENTS

4 cups plain Greek yogurt, divided

1 cup sliced strawberries, divided

6 tablespoons chopped walnuts, divided

8 teaspoons low-carb pancake syrup

DIRECTIONS

1 Place ½ cup of yogurt into four bowls.

2 Top each with ¼ cup sliced strawberries and 1 tablespoon of the chopped walnuts.

3 Drizzle the strawberries with 1 teaspoon of the pancake syrup.

4 Add another ½ cup of yogurt to each bowl.

5 Sprinkle the remaining walnuts on top of each parfait and drizzle with another teaspoon of pancake syrup. Enjoy!

PER SERVING: *Calories 335; Fat 22g; Cholesterol 38mg; Sodium 135mg; Carbohydrate 19g (Dietary Fiber 5g, Sugar Alcohol 2g); Net Carbohydrate 13g; Protein 23g.*

Chocolate Cheesecake Dip with Strawberries

PREP TIME: 10 MIN	COOK TIME: 2 MIN	YIELD: 4 SERVINGS

INGREDIENTS

4 ounces Lily's chocolate chips

8 ounces cream cheese (1 cup)

½ cup powdered erythritol

2 tablespoons butter

1½ teaspoons vanilla extract

1 cup heavy cream

16 ounces strawberries (1 pound)

DIRECTIONS

1 Place the chocolate chips in a microwave-safe bowl. Microwave on high, heating and stirring in 30-second increments until the chocolate is melted.

2 In a separate bowl, mix together the cream cheese, erythritol, butter, and vanilla until smooth. Fold in the melted chocolate.

3 Slowly pour in the heavy cream, beating the mixture until it is stiff.

4 Refrigerate the dip for about 30 minutes to let it set.

5 Dip fresh strawberries (or eat it by the spoonful!) and enjoy.

PER SERVING: *Calories 592; Fat 57g; Cholesterol 159mg; Sodium 232mg; Carbohydrate 55g (Dietary Fiber 10g, Sugar Alcohol 30g); Net Carbohydrate 15g; Protein 7g.*

Lemon Ricotta Waffles with Ice Cream

PREP TIME: 5 MIN	COOK TIME: 10 MIN	YIELD: 4 SERVINGS

INGREDIENTS

4 large eggs

1 cup whole milk ricotta cheese

¼ cup heavy cream

1 tablespoon vanilla extract

1 tablespoon lemon zest

2 tablespoons granulated erythritol

6 tablespoons coconut flour

¼ cup almond flour

½ teaspoon baking soda

2 tablespoons butter, divided

1 cup vanilla keto ice cream, divided

Chopped almonds and unsweetened shredded coconut (optional)

DIRECTIONS

1 Place the eggs, ricotta, heavy cream, vanilla, lemon zest, erythritol, coconut flour, almond flour, and baking soda in a large bowl and whisk everything together until smooth.

2 Use a silicon brush to grease your waffle iron with the butter. (Don't use the 2 tablespoons all at once; rather, spread it out among the batches of waffles.)

3 Heat your waffle maker according to the manufacturer's directions.

4 Pour about 1 cup of batter into the waffle iron, close, and bake. The amount of batter will vary based on your waffle maker; check the manufacturer's directions to find the recommended quantity of batter.

5 Once the waffles are golden brown and crisp, remove them from the waffle iron and place them on a plate. Repeat until you've used up all the batter.

6 Add a scoop of keto ice cream on top of the warm waffle. Sprinkle with chopped almonds and shredded coconut if desired. Enjoy right away!

PER SERVING: *Calories 459; Fat 35g; Cholesterol 230mg; Sodium 314mg; Carbohydrate 24g (Dietary Fiber 8g, Sugar Alcohol 8g); Net Carbohydrate 8g; Protein 20g.*

Almond Pound Cake

PREP TIME: 10 MIN | **COOK TIME: 35 MIN** | **YIELD: 12 SERVINGS**

INGREDIENTS

3 large eggs

½ cup granular erythritol

⅓ cup unsweetened almond milk

2 teaspoons baking powder

1 tablespoon almond extract

¼ teaspoon salt

½ cup butter, melted

2½ cups almond flour

½ cup sliced almonds

DIRECTIONS

1 Preheat the oven to 325 degrees and grease an 8-inch springform pan with butter.

2 In a large bowl, beat the eggs, erythritol, almond milk, baking powder, almond extract, and salt.

3 Pour the melted butter into the batter while beating.

4 Add the almond flour and stir into a thick batter.

5 Pour the batter into the prepared pan and bake for 35 minutes.

6 Remove the cake from the oven and sprinkle the almond slices over the top right away.

7 Let the cake cool and then slice and serve.

PER SERVING: *Calories 251; Fat 23g; Cholesterol 60mg; Sodium 130mg; Carbohydrate 14g (Dietary Fiber 3g, Sugar Alcohol 8g); Net Carbohydrate 3g; Protein 8g.*

6

The Part of Tens

Find out which health conditions the keto diet helps the most.

Discover some famous names who have tried and loved keto.

Know the value of maximizing healthy fats in your diet.

Chapter 26

Ten Health Conditions that Can Benefit from Keto

A keto diet can greatly impact many aspects of your health. People turn to the keto diet for weight loss, blood-sugar control, and to help boost energy levels. It can help you sleep better, improve your skin clarity, and even help prevent neurodegenerative diseases. The keto diet is more than just a simple diet that limits carbs, it is a complete way of life that helps you live happier and healthier.

In this chapter we talk a little about the top ten health conditions that can benefit from a keto diet. You will be amazed when you discover how many ailments can be lessened, controlled, or even cured through keto.

Type 2 Diabetes

Type 2 diabetes is the first condition many people think of when they assess the benefits of the keto diet. Many studies have shown that a very low-carb diet helps regulate blood-sugar levels. People with type 2 diabetes show reduced blood-sugar levels when they switch to a keto diet. Many people with type 2 diabetes can reduce their dosage of medication and manage their blood sugar easily when following a strict low-carb diet. People even report eliminating medication altogether and controlling their diabetes with diet alone.

When you eat carbs and sugars, your blood sugar levels rise rapidly and crash just as quickly. People with diabetes have a very hard time processing sugars, which can cause blood-sugar levels to remain dangerously high or, on the other end of the spectrum, crash extremely low. When you switch to a keto diet, your body no longer needs to tackle the spikes of your blood-sugar levels after you eat carbs, and insulin sensitivity gets restored.

A keto diet can help those with diabetes reduce their blood-sugar levels and return them to normal. Keto food is much easier to process for anyone with diabetes, and notice that the positive effects can be seen almost instantly.

Epilepsy

The keto diet was first tested in a health setting in the 1920s when it was used to help children with epilepsy. Epilepsy is a disease that causes seizures due to high levels of brain activity. The keto diet works to control epilepsy by altering how the brain gets its energy to function. Rather than using carbs as fuel, it processes ketones created from fats. The lower blood-sugar levels and fats as fuel reduce the excitability of the brain and, therefore, lower the tendency for the brain to generate seizures.

Studies have shown that more than half of children who suffer from epilepsy benefit from a keto diet. About 20 percent of children reportedly achieve a 90 percent reduction in seizures. This is an incredibly high number for such a simple dietary switch. You can see why doctors suggest a keto diet to control epilepsy.

Obesity

Obesity is a major health condition that affects millions of people in the United States alone. About 2 in every 5 adults have obesity, and 1 in every 11 adults have severe obesity. Obesity can lead to many other health concerns caused by excess weight. Type 2 diabetes, heart disease, high cholesterol, and arthritis are just a few conditions that can be directly linked to obesity.

Not only does the keto diet limit carb intake, but it also puts your body into fat-burning mode. Studies have shown that diets limiting carbs are far more effective weight-loss tools than diets that restrict calories. Keto diets are satiating and filling while also helping you lose weight.

Polycystic Ovarian Syndrome

Polycystic ovarian syndrome, also known as PCOS, is a hormonal condition that can result in infertility or irregular periods in women. Other side effects of PCOS include obesity, insulin resistance, acne, and excess facial hair.

The keto diet has been shown to help those with PCOS by lowering and stabilizing blood-sugar levels. There is lots of anecdotal evidence from people who suffer from PCOS and try a keto diet. They can lose weight quickly and lower insulin levels. Some have even found the keto diet to help improve fertility.

Autism

Autism and epilepsy both can cause overactivity in the brain, which leads to seizures. Therefore, many doctors feel the keto diet can help those with autism, just as it has helped reduce seizure activity caused by epilepsy. The keto diet can reduce brain cell overstimulation, and it has also been shown to benefit behavioral health as well.

Autism typically creates issues with social interaction and communication. Studies have shown that a cyclical keto diet can help improve autism spectrum disorder behavior patterns. A *cyclical keto diet* involves one or two days a week of carb-loading and the other five or six days staying under 30 grams of net carbs per day. A gluten-free keto diet has also been shown to be beneficial.

Multiple Sclerosis

Multiple sclerosis (MS) is caused by damage to the nerves in the brain, which results in communication problems between the body and the brain. Those with MS may have difficulty controlling their body and have challenges when it comes to balancing, general movement, memory, and vision.

The keto diet can help reduce inflammation in the brain and body. Reduced inflammation can lead to improved memory and physical activity. The keto diet also switches the body from sourcing energy from sugar to getting energy from ketones made from fat. Studies have found that those with MS have an easier time processing ketones than sugar as a source of fuel. Those who tried a keto diet had more energy and were able to function with more ease.

Metabolic Syndrome

Metabolic syndrome is also known as prediabetes. The body is resistant to insulin and has an increased risk of heart disease. High blood pressure, elevated triglycerides, and extreme weight gain are all symptoms of metabolic syndrome. The keto diet has been shown to help improve all these side effects and greatly help those with metabolic syndrome.

Many studies have shown that the keto diet helps improve cholesterol, lower blood pressure, and greatly reduce blood-sugar levels. When these health issues are fixed, or at least improved, the symptoms of metabolic syndrome are also improved.

In one study, participants with metabolic syndrome who switched to a keto diet were able to lower body fat, decrease triglycerides, lower blood-pressure levels, and lower blood sugar. All these improvements made the participants feel better and function more easily. The keto diet has a huge positive impact on metabolic syndrome, and many doctors are turning toward prescribing a keto lifestyle rather than medication to improve this health issue.

Traumatic Brain Injury

Traumatic brain injury (TBI) is caused by an intense head injury, typically from a car accident or severe fall. A brain injury can have long-term, damaging effects on memory, personality, and the body's overall ability to function. Injured brain cells don't recover as easily as other cells in the body, which means those who suffer from TBI are likely to experience the negative consequences of the injury long term.

Researchers believe that those who have TBI may benefit from the keto diet primarily because of the diet's anti-inflammatory effects. The keto diet can help reduce swelling in the brain, which can improve motor function and memory.

Ketones are also a more accessible source of energy than sugar for fueling the brain. Those with TBI may be able to process ketones better than they are able to process sugar.

Animal studies have shown that the keto diet does benefit those suffering from TBI, but more studies need to be done on humans to determine the true results.

Alzheimer's Disease

Alzheimer's disease is a severe form of dementia that can impair memory, both long- and short-term. It is caused by plaque buildup in the brain, neurofibrillary tangles, and shrinkage in the posterior part of the brain. Those who have Alzheimer's disease are unable to use glucose as an energy source properly and may suffer from inflammation linked to insulin resistance.

Several studies on animals have shown that a ketogenic diet can help improve balance and coordination in those with Alzheimer's. The keto diet reduces inflammation, which may help improve overall brain function.

Supplementing a keto diet with ketone esters showed a reduced brain plaque buildup. A study found that those who took an MCT compound while also following a keto diet had greatly improved mental functions. More studies are currently being done to see how ketone esters work to help those with Alzheimer's disease, and the results are already promising.

Migraine Headaches

About one billion people around the world suffer from migraine headaches. Migraines involve severe pain, nausea, and sensitivity to light. Many people who have chronic migraines report that standard pain medication does not help reduce the symptoms.

Studies suggest that a ketogenic diet may help lessen, if not eliminate, migraines. The keto diet can reduce inflammation in the brain, which is typically a source of migraines. With less inflammation, the pain caused by a migraine also decreases. Some who followed a strict keto diet reported a significant decrease in migraines. More scientific studies are needed to make conclusive statements, but the evidence so far points to the keto diet significantly reducing migraines.

Chapter **27**

Ten Celebrities Who Swear by Keto

Thousands and thousands of people swear by the keto diet, but it's celebrities who really bring the diet into the public eye. Many celebrities have tried the keto diet and discovered its true power. Their keto journeys have helped many others find the keto path.

Here are some popular celebrities who have turned to the keto diet. If you are also inspired by celebrities and interested in their successes, you'll be even more motivated to start on a keto diet after reading these stories.

Halle Berry

Halle Berry is one of the original celebrities to try the keto diet. She has been following the diet for years, even before it became a trend. Berry started her keto diet to help control her type 2 diabetes. She was diagnosed with the health condition when she was only 22 years old, and a low-carb diet was recommended to help her manage her condition. As you know, the keto diet can help control blood-sugar levels and those with diabetes greatly.

Berry likes to refer to keto as a "lifestyle change" rather than solely a diet. Not only does it help her manage her diabetes, but she also says keto is responsible for helping her lose weight after having a baby, boosting her overall energy levels, and improving her mental performance. She even says the keto diet helped slow down the aging process, helping her look and feel better despite getting older. Halle Berry is a big keto fan!

Megan Fox

Megan Fox has also been following the keto diet for years. She is very strict about the no-carb rules and claims she never has cheat days. The actress has said that once she committed to keto, she never considered eating carbs again. She even claims to be repulsed by bread.

Fox says that eating carbs didn't make her feel good, so she completely cut out pretzels, chips, crackers, and fruits that didn't fit into her diet plan. It took her body about a week to adjust, and then she felt great. Fox says the keto diet and long walks are what help keep her fit and in shape. Even after having three kids, Megan Fox is looking as good as ever!

Vanessa Hudgens

Some Hollywood roles require actors to gain weight to play a certain part. This is what happened to Vanessa Hudgens when she starred in the movie *Gimme Shelter*. After gaining 20 pounds for the role, Hudgens was eager to lose weight, so she turned to the keto diet.

Hudgens eats lots of eggs, bacon, avocadoes, and greens throughout the day. She likes to snack on nuts and keto-friendly fruits, and then have steak or salmon for dinner. She openly talks about how fats make you feel fuller for longer and therefore help you lose weight.

The actress also practices intermittent fasting, which helps her feel more powerful during her workouts. Hudgens says she loves the keto diet because she gets the nutrients she needs and gets to eat what she wants.

Kourtney Kardashian

The Kardashian sisters have promoted many different diets over the years, but Kourtney seems to be a big fan of the keto diet. She often talks about following a gluten-free, sugar-free style of eating that fits right into the keto guidelines. She has even discussed how she tries to stay in ketosis so her body will burn fat for energy.

Kourtney wrote on her website about her low-carb detox dietary plan. A green smoothie, an avocado, and some lean protein and veggies are highlighted as her daily choices. She even adds MCT oil to her smoothies to boost the fat and help give her more energy. Her website features the exact keto meals she likes to eat, so if you're interested in following the Kardashian keto plan, you can check it out.

Adriana Lima

Being a supermodel means staying in shape to look your best. That's why Adriana Lima turned to a keto lifestyle. The model sticks to a strict no-carb policy, avoiding even carrots to keep carbs at bay.

Lima says she first turned to the keto diet to lose a few pounds for the Victoria's Secret Show; however, she loved how keto eating made her feel and look. If she eats carbs now, she feels "swollen." So, it's chicken, green veggies, and protein shakes for this supermodel, and it's working great for her.

Tim Tebow

The former NFL quarterback and current TV sports anchor is a big fan of the keto lifestyle. This shows that even athletes can use keto to provide them with plenty of energy to do all the things they love.

Tebow likes to start the day with a fat-filled coffee. He uses half decaf, half regular coffee mixed with some heavy cream, almond milk, stevia, and Kerrygold butter. Talk about waking up with a delicious dose of fats! After his morning coffee, Tebow likes to eat eggs, yogurt, lean meats, and lots of guacamole.

Tebow tries to keep his macros at 75 percent fats, 20 percent protein, and 5 percent carbs. However, he also loves the keto diet because you can just eat until you are full without worrying about counting calories. Once you follow the keto diet for a while, you naturally know which foods give you the most energy.

Katie Couric

The former *Today Show* anchor tried the keto diet and was very open about her experiences. She posted her keto journey on Instagram and said that she struggled in the beginning. The fourth and fifth days of keto were hard due to the keto flu, which is unfortunately typical. But once she got past those rough days, Couric said she felt much better. She was enjoying putting half-and-half in her coffee and getting extra fats into her system.

While Couric did not stick to the keto diet long-term, she did claim to feel good while on the keto diet. The keto lifestyle is a big commitment, and it isn't for everyone. But even those who don't stay with keto see how it can be beneficial. You never know until you try!

Lebron James

Lebron James claims that the keto diet helped him lose a ton of weight. The NBA superstar tried the keto diet for 67 days to slim down and get back in shape. He cut out sugar, carbs, and all dairy (which we don't recommend, but it is an option).

Not only did James lose weight, but he also improved his performance on the court. The keto diet is known to help you have excess, sustained energy. The body functions better when it uses fats as fuel rather than quickly burning through carbs and then crashing. James also wanted the mental focus that keto can bring.

Al Roker

Al Roker is a well-known TV personality who lost a significant amount of weight in 2018. How did he lose over 40 pounds? By sticking to a keto diet. Not only did Roker lose lots of weight through the keto diet, but he is also controlling his cholesterol levels thanks to keto.

Roker posts his favorite keto recipes and creations often on his Instagram account. He has even made some of his favorite keto meals on TV. While Roker is a big fan of the keto diet, he doesn't push his dietary beliefs on his loyal followers. He has said, "What works for you, works for you." But his success even made his TV co-star Savannah Guthrie try keto as well. Seems like keto is a trend going around the *TODAY* show set!

Vinny Guadagnino

The *Jersey Shore* star gave the keto diet a try and lost over 50 pounds. He became a big supporter of the keto diet and posts keto tips on his Instagram (aptly named @KetoGuido) page regularly. His biggest tip is to not overthink it and take the keto diet one meal at a time.

Guadagnino says that when you are hungry, your brain is more tempted to want junk food and quick, unhealthy carbs. When you are satiated and full, you are more likely to think rationally. This is why he says snacking (on keto foods, of course!) is so important to him. Avoiding hunger pangs helps you make better food choices.

Chapter **28**

Ten Benefits of Eating Healthy Fats

We talk a lot about the benefits of fats throughout this book. We go into lots of detail about why fats are good and not as harmful as you may have been led to believe. Fats are good!

For years, we have been led to believe that fats are evil. We have been taught that fat can raise cholesterol, and increase the chances of heart disease and obesity. However, scientific research now shows that there are so many amazing benefits to eating more fat. We all need to rethink this essential part of our diet and open our eyes to how great fats can be.

We want to give you a very clear view of the benefits of fats, so here are ten benefits of eating healthy fats, easily laid out and explained. You will be a believer in fats soon enough.

Fat Is Essential to Brain Health

The brain is made up of almost 60 percent fat. You need to consume fats for your brain to function well. When you follow a low-fat diet, you rob your brain of the nutrients it needs to function properly.

In addition to needing fat to help cellular regeneration, the brain also needs fats to get essential vitamins and minerals. Vitamins A, D, E, and K are not water-soluble vitamins. This means that fats must be transported to the brain and absorbed. Without fats as carriers, these vitamins can't be used by the body and just pass right through the digestive system.

Vitamin D is an essential nutrient for the brain and has been linked to decreasing the probability of Alzheimer's disease, Parkinson's disease, and other cognitive functions.

Fats Boost the Immune System

You may already know that vitamin C and antioxidants can help boost the immune system. Did you know that fats also improve immunity?

When white blood cells don't have enough fatty acids, they are unable to recognize foreign invaders like bacteria and viruses. When the white blood cells are weak and unable to do their job, you are more likely to get sick.

Saturated fats like butter and coconut oil have been shown to help improve immunity. They help white blood cells stay healthy, strong, and able to fight off illness.

Promote Skin Health

Most of our cellular membrane is made from fats. Your largest organ, your skin, is made up of millions and millions of cells. This means that your skin is made primarily from fats.

Consuming healthy fats helps prevent your skin from being too dry or chapped. Think about how you rub lotion over your body when your skin feels dry. What are you putting on your skin? Fats! Compared to applying fats to your skin externally, eating enough healthy fats and healing your skin from the inside out is better.

Dry, damaged skin is not only uncomfortable but also bad for your health. Cracked skin can allow germs and infections into your system, making you sick much more easily. Eating healthy fats keeps your biggest organ healthy, strong, and feeling good.

Fats Help Cholesterol

For many years, we have thought that fats raise cholesterol levels. While eating lots of fats can increase cholesterol, it is HDL, the "good kind" of cholesterol, that is affected and increased. Higher levels of HDL have an anti-inflammatory effect and are also antimicrobial. You want your HDL to be raised and your LDL to be lowered. Eating healthy fats can help accomplish this.

Scientists recommend incorporating healthy fats into your diet. Eating mackerel, salmon, olive oil, and avocados can reduce cholesterol levels. Polyunsaturated fats give your body nutrients while keeping your cholesterol levels under control.

Increase Muscle Mass

Adding beneficial fats to your diet can help balance your hormones and improve recovery after an intense workout. In fact, sports nutrition researchers have found that a higher fat intake can not only increase muscle gain but also decrease inflammation.

Consuming more fats helps you recover quickly from a workout and helps your muscles rebuild in a healthy, strong way. Omega-3 fatty acids are the best when it comes to improving muscle, but MCT oil (medium-chain triglycerides) can be just as beneficial. If you are looking to add muscle, eating fats and more protein is a great way to do it.

Reduce Risk of Cancer

Eating "good" fats can help decrease inflammation and reduce the risk of certain cancers. Research has shown that monounsaturated fats, like those found in olive oil, have a protective effect and can help guard cells from metastasis.

Omega-3 fats have the biggest impact on preventing cancer. They have potent anti-inflammatory effects that can guard against cancer cells. Studies have even shown that an increased intake of omega-3 fats is associated with a 41 percent reduced risk of colorectal cancer. These fats have also been shown to reduce the risk of breast cancer. A separate study showed that men who consumed fish five times a week reduced the risk of death from prostate cancer by almost half. Omega-3 fatty acids are amazing when it comes to helping prevent cancer. These are statistics you don't see from carbs!

Develop Strong Bones

We talk earlier in this chapter about how fat is needed to help the body absorb some vitamins. Vitamin K is a perfect example of a fat-soluble vitamin that requires dietary fats to be utilized inside the body.

Vitamin K is one of the key vitamins your body needs to improve bone strength. Vitamins K, D, and A (all fat-soluble) work together with calcium and magnesium to solidify and harden bones. Monounsaturated fats have been shown to be the most beneficial when it comes to bone health. They reduce oxidative stress and inflammation while delivering vitamins and minerals to the body. Polyunsaturated fats are also beneficial to bone health. However, omega-6 fatty acids may contribute to bone density loss. It is essential to know which fats are beneficial and which are harmful. Stay focused on healthy fats as they are more abundant and the benefits are much greater.

Rapid Weight Loss

Eating more fats may help you lose weight. So many dieters try to avoid fats, but this isn't the way to reach weight-loss goals. In fact, carbs are the biggest contributor to weight gain, not fat. When you opt for a low-fat diet, you are automatically going to increase your carb intake, which then causes you to gain weight.

Eating a diet full of healthy fats can help promote satiety, making you feel fuller for longer. This decreases your food intake in general and helps you consume less food in a pleasant, easy way.

When your body is in ketosis, you are burning fats in your body to use as energy. The ketogenic diet has shown that increasing fat intake helps you burn fat, reduce fat stores in the body, and increase your metabolic rate. All these changes help you lose weight quickly and efficiently. The best part is that you get to enjoy incredible food while you do it!

Fats May Prevent Heart Disease

Saturated fats are often linked to heart disease; however, it's not that simple. Healthy fats can help combat that problem and even reduce the risk of heart disease.

Omega-6 fatty acids have been shown to help reduce the risk of heart disease while consuming carbs makes heart disease more likely. Olive oil, nut oils, avocados, and fish oils are good choices for a heart-healthy diet. Adding ground flaxseeds to your diet is an easy way to get more fiber and omega-3 fatty acids, both of which have heart-healthy effects. These foods have saturated fats in them but in a limited quantity, and the saturated fats all come from whole foods. Saturated fat from fast-food meals and processed foods are the ones you want to watch out for.

The key is to know which fats are good for your heart and which ones are problematic. Once you understand this, you will know which fats help improve your heart.

Improve Eye Health

Omega-3 fatty acids have so many benefits, including improved eye health. They have been linked to preventing dry eyes and help ensure the eye drains fluids correctly. Getting enough omega-3 in your diet can help prevent glaucoma and even reduce retina deterioration.

You can boost your omega-3 intake by eating fish, taking fish oil supplements, adding flaxseed to your diet, or eating nuts like walnuts. Getting the proper amount of omega-3 fatty acids is essential to eye health. Just another reason why your body needs fats to function properly.

Metric Conversion Guide

Note: The recipes in this book weren't developed or tested using metric measurements. There may be some variation in quality when converting to metric units.

Common Abbreviations

Abbreviation(s)	What It Stands For
cm	Centimeter
C., c.	Cup
G, g	Gram
kg	Kilogram
L, l	Liter
lb.	Pound
mL, ml	Milliliter
oz.	Ounce
pt.	Pint
t., tsp.	Teaspoon
T., Tb., Tbsp.	Tablespoon

Volume

U.S. Units	Canadian Metric	Australian Metric
¼ teaspoon	1 milliliter	1 milliliter
½ teaspoon	2 milliliters	2 milliliters
1 teaspoon	5 milliliters	5 milliliters
1 tablespoon	15 milliliters	20 milliliters
¼ cup	50 milliliters	60 milliliters
⅓ cup	75 milliliters	80 milliliters
½ cup	125 milliliters	125 milliliters
⅔ cup	150 milliliters	170 milliliters
¾ cup	175 milliliters	190 milliliters
1 cup	250 milliliters	250 milliliters
1 quart	1 liter	1 liter
1½ quarts	1.5 liters	1.5 liters
2 quarts	2 liters	2 liters
2½ quarts	2.5 liters	2.5 liters
3 quarts	3 liters	3 liters
4 quarts (1 gallon)	4 liters	4 liters

Weight

U.S. Units	Canadian Metric	Australian Metric
1 ounce	30 grams	30 grams
2 ounces	55 grams	60 grams
3 ounces	85 grams	90 grams
4 ounces (¼ pound)	115 grams	125 grams
8 ounces (½ pound)	225 grams	225 grams
16 ounces (1 pound)	455 grams	500 grams (½ kilogram)

Length

Inches	Centimeters
0.5	1.5
1	2.5
2	5.0
3	7.5
4	10.0
5	12.5
6	15.0
7	17.5
8	20.5
9	23.0
10	25.5
11	28.0
12	30.5

Temperature (Degrees)

Fahrenheit	Celsius
32	0
212	100
250	120
275	140
300	150
325	160
350	180
375	190
400	200
425	220
450	230
475	240
500	260

Index

About the Authors

Rami and Vicky Abrams are two entrepreneurs based in Brooklyn, New York. They first discovered the keto diet in 2014 and were initially (and understandably) a little skeptical about a diet that allowed more butter and bacon intake than it did whole grains. Never ones to live with unsatisfied curiosity, they dug deep into the diet's background. They were impressed by its foundation as a peer-reviewed medical treatment and weight-loss tool and decided to give it a shot. Within a few weeks, they were steadily moving toward their goal weights and had never felt better.

Seeing the scale move in the right direction, seemingly effortlessly, was great. Still, the two most significant advantages they noticed were a steady energy state and increased mental clarity throughout the day. The further they traveled on their keto journey, the more consistent and energetic they felt; what started as a short-term experiment turned into a complete life transformation.

Rami and Vicky are self-professed "foodies" who love trying new dishes and genres at every opportunity. Although enthralled with their new way of "fat-focused" cooking with all the flavors it provided, the couple found that they were missing many of their old favorites. Determined to have their cake and eat it, too, they began to seek new ways of re-creating established conventions in the kitchen.

It involved a few trials and errors (and several unfortunate encounters with the smoke detector), but eventually, they experienced a breakthrough. Vicky is fond of saying there are ways to re-create almost all your favorite foods, including desserts. A diet that eliminates sugar and other harmful sweeteners is quite an achievement!

At the beginning of 2015, Rami and Vicky developed Tasteaholics.com and focused on writing research-heavy articles while creating and photographing recipes and blogging about their progress. The site rapidly became renowned as an expert source for keto information and tantalizing recipes. By the second year, they began publishing their popular cookbook series called *Keto in Five*. The cookbooks center on three basic principles: Every dish contains five or fewer grams of net carbs per serving, is made with up to five ingredients, and can be prepared in five easy steps. Their efforts were so successful that they quit their jobs and focused exclusively on Tasteaholics.

In 2017, the Abrams launched So Nourished, Inc., a company dedicated to creating low-carb ingredients and products, such as healthy sugar replacements and low-carb brownies, pancake mixes, and syrups. They also expanded their sites to include meal plans and keto news articles, and they launched the Total Keto Diet mobile app.

The Total Keto Diet App allows users to track their meals and exercise and automatically generate weekly meal plans for each user based on their specific dietary needs and preferences.

Although they stay busy, the Abrams found plenty of time to engage in two of their favorite activities: traveling and trying new food. In one year, they spent six months exploring eight different countries, sampling each area's delicacies, and blogging about the keto lifestyle and low-carb recipes from around the globe.

As the healthy fat revolution continues, Rami and Vicky remain dedicated to spreading the word about the benefits of ketosis in every area of life.

Dedication

To our low-carb family at large: You inspire us every day. From the energy you display on social media, which fuels our innovation, to the encouragement we regularly find in our inboxes, you've become a family we never knew we needed. Thank you for bucking tradition with us, being willing to ask questions and explore new territory, and relentlessly demanding health *and* flavor!

Authors' Acknowledgments

In writing this book, we are indebted to numerous experts, researchers, and fellow low-carb pioneers who have tirelessly worked to discover the truth.

Our dear friend, Yuriy Petriv, was our earliest keto diet influencer, introducing us not only to the ketogenic lifestyle but also to each other! His friendship and partnership (in So Nourished, Inc.) have been the cornerstones of our personal and business efforts from the beginning.

Writing this book would not have been possible without Tracy Boggier, senior acquisitions editor at Wiley, who brought this project to us. We want to thank the entire team of editors who worked on this book: Donna Wright (project editor), Christine Pingleton (copy editor), and Emily Nolan (recipe tester).

Publisher's Acknowledgments

Senior Acquisitions Editor: Tracy Boggier

Project Editor: Donna Wright

Copy Editor: Christine Pingleton

Recipe Tester: Emily Nolan

Photographers: Wendy Jo Peterson and Grace Geri Goodale

Production Editor: Tamilmani Varadharaj

Back Cover Image: Courtesy of Wendy Jo Peterson and Grace Geri Goodale

Take dummies with you everywhere you go!

Whether you are excited about e-books, want more from the web, must have your mobile apps, or are swept up in social media, dummies makes everything easier.

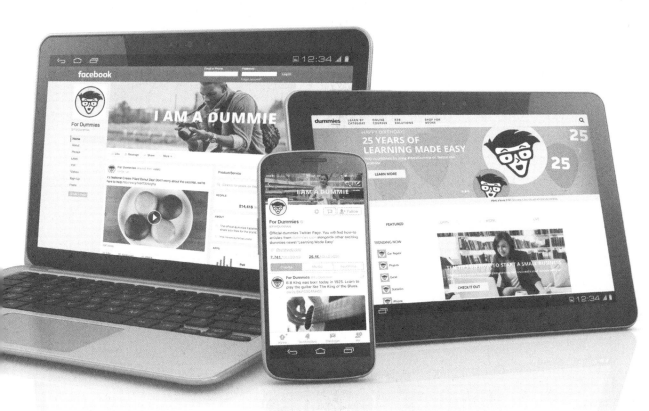

Find us online!

dummies.com

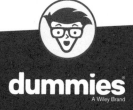

Leverage the power

Dummies is the global leader in the reference category and one of the most trusted and highly regarded brands in the world. No longer just focused on books, customers now have access to the dummies content they need in the format they want. Together we'll craft a solution that engages your customers, stands out from the competition, and helps you meet your goals.

Advertising & Sponsorships

Connect with an engaged audience on a powerful multimedia site, and position your message alongside expert how-to content. Dummies.com is a one-stop shop for free, online information and know-how curated by a team of experts.

- Targeted ads
- Video
- Email Marketing
- Microsites
- Sweepstakes sponsorship

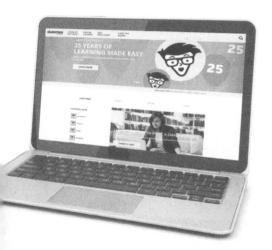

20 MILLION PAGE VIEWS EVERY SINGLE MONTH

15 MILLION UNIQUE VISITORS PER MONTH

43% OF ALL VISITORS ACCESS THE SITE VIA THEIR MOBILE DEVICES

700,000 NEWSLETTER SUBSCRIPTIONS TO THE INBOXES OF *300,000* UNIQUE INDIVIDUALS EVERY WEEK

# of dummies

Custom Publishing

Reach a global audience in any language by creating a solution that will differentiate you from competitors, amplify your message, and encourage customers to make a buying decision.

- Apps
- Books
- eBooks
- Video
- Audio
- Webinars

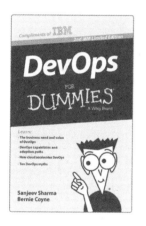
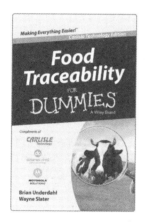
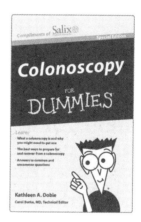
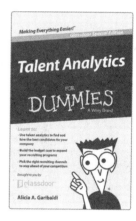

Brand Licensing & Content

Leverage the strength of the world's most popular reference brand to reach new audiences and channels of distribution.

For more information, visit **dummies.com/biz**

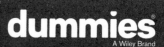

dummies®
A Wiley Brand

PERSONAL ENRICHMENT

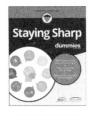

9781119187790
USA $26.00
CAN $31.99
UK £19.99

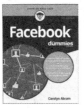

9781119179030
USA $21.99
CAN $25.99
UK £16.99

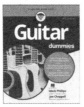

9781119293354
USA $24.99
CAN $29.99
UK £17.99

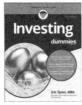

9781119293347
USA $22.99
CAN $27.99
UK £16.99

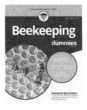

9781119310068
USA $22.99
CAN $27.99
UK £16.99

9781119235606
USA $24.99
CAN $29.99
UK £17.99

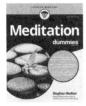

9781119251163
USA $24.99
CAN $29.99
UK £17.99

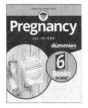

9781119235491
USA $26.99
CAN $31.99
UK £19.99

9781119279952
USA $24.99
CAN $29.99
UK £17.99

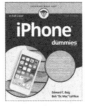

9781119283133
USA $24.99
CAN $29.99
UK £17.99

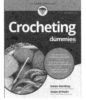

9781119287117
USA $24.99
CAN $29.99
UK £16.99

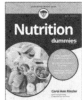

9781119130246
USA $22.99
CAN $27.99
UK £16.99

PROFESSIONAL DEVELOPMENT

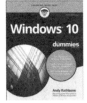

9781119311041
USA $24.99
CAN $29.99
UK £17.99

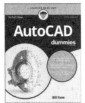

9781119255796
USA $39.99
CAN $47.99
UK £27.99

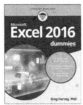

9781119293439
USA $26.99
CAN $31.99
UK £19.99

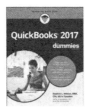

9781119281467
USA $26.99
CAN $31.99
UK £19.99

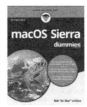

9781119280651
USA $29.99
CAN $35.99
UK £21.99

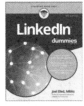

9781119251132
USA $24.99
CAN $29.99
UK £17.99

9781119310563
USA $34.00
CAN $41.99
UK £24.99

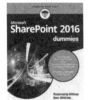

9781119181705
USA $29.99
CAN $35.99
UK £21.99

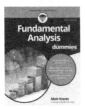

9781119263593
USA $26.99
CAN $31.99
UK £19.99

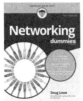

9781119257769
USA $29.99
CAN $35.99
UK £21.99

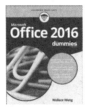

9781119293477
USA $26.99
CAN $31.99
UK £19.99

9781119265313
USA $24.99
CAN $29.99
UK £17.99

9781119239314
USA $29.99
CAN $35.99
UK £21.99

9781119293323
USA $29.99
CAN $35.99
UK £21.99

dummies.com

dummies
A Wiley Brand

Learning Made Easy

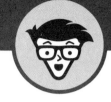

ACADEMIC

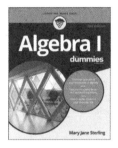

9781119293576
USA $19.99
CAN $23.99
UK £15.99

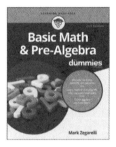

9781119293637
USA $19.99
CAN $23.99
UK £15.99

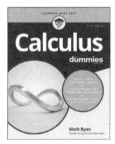

9781119293491
USA $19.99
CAN $23.99
UK £15.99

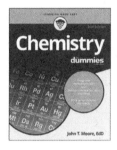

9781119293460
USA $19.99
CAN $23.99
UK £15.99

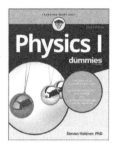

9781119293590
USA $19.99
CAN $23.99
UK £15.99

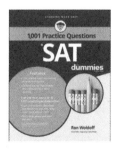

9781119215844
USA $26.99
CAN $31.99
UK £19.99

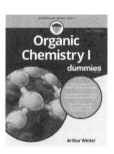

9781119293378
USA $22.99
CAN $27.99
UK £16.99

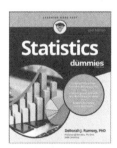

9781119293521
USA $19.99
CAN $23.99
UK £15.99

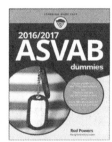

9781119239178
USA $18.99
CAN $22.99
UK £14.99

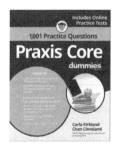

9781119263883
USA $26.99
CAN $31.99
UK £19.99

Available Everywhere Books Are Sold

dummies.com

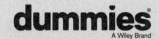

Small books for big imaginations

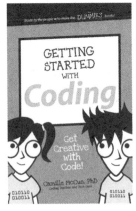

9781119177173
USA $9.99
CAN $9.99
UK £8.99

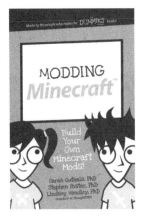

9781119177272
USA $9.99
CAN $9.99
UK £8.99

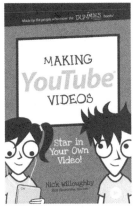

9781119177241
USA $9.99
CAN $9.99
UK £8.99

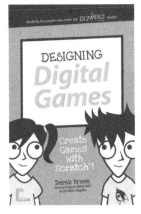

9781119177210
USA $9.99
CAN $9.99
UK £8.99

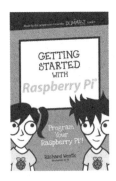

9781119262657
USA $9.99
CAN $9.99
UK £6.99

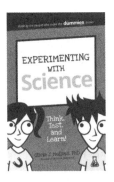

9781119291336
USA $9.99
CAN $9.99
UK £6.99

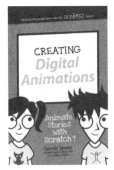

9781119233527
USA $9.99
CAN $9.99
UK £6.99

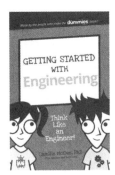

9781119291220
USA $9.99
CAN $9.99
UK £6.99

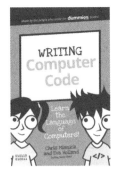

9781119177302
USA $9.99
CAN $9.99
UK £8.99

Unleash Their Creativity

dummies.com

dummies
A Wiley Brand